MUSCLE MEDICINE

THE REVOLUTIONARY APPROACH TO MAINTAINING, STRENGTHENING, AND REPAIRING YOUR MUSCLES AND JOINTS

Rob DeStefano, D.C., with Bryan Kelly, M.D.
and Joseph Hooper

A FIRESIDE BOOK
Published by Simon & Schuster
New York London Toronto Sydney

Fireside
A Division of Simon & Schuster, Inc.
1230 Avenue of the Americas
New York, NY 10020

For information about special discounts for bulk purchases,
please contact Simon & Schuster Special Sales at
1-866-506-1949 or business@simonandschuster.com

The Simon & Schuster Speakers Bureau can bring authors to your
live event. For more information or to book an event contact the
Simon & Schuster Speakers Bureau at 1-866-248-3049 or visit our
website at www.simonspeakers.com.

Designed by Ruth Lee-Mui
Photographs by Brooke & Eric Lagstein of Be Creative Photography
Illustrations by Karen Kuchar and Dr. Rob DeStefano

Manufactured in the United States of America

10 9 8 7 6 5 4 3

Library of Congress Cataloging-in-Publication Data
DeStefano, Rob.
   Muscle medicine : the revolutionary approach to maintaining, strengthening,
and repairing your muscles and joints / Rob DeStefano with Bryan Kelly ;
and Joseph Hooper.—1st Fireside trade pbk. ed.
      p.   cm.
   Includes bibliographical references and index.
   1. Muscles—Physiology.   2. Muscles—Metabolism.   3. Muscles—
Regeneration.   I. Kelly, Bryan.   II. Hooper, Joseph.   III. Title.
   QP321.D375   2009
   612.7'4—dc22   2009007183

ISBN 978-1-4165-6256-6
ISBN 978-1-4165-6278-8 (eBook)

To Ronnie Barnes, Dr. Russell Warren,
The New York Football Giants,
and all of our athletes and patients,
thank you.

CONTENTS

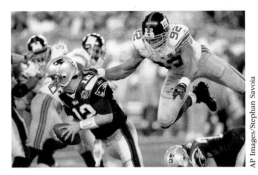

AP Images/Stephan Savoia

FOREWORD

by Michael Strahan

It's a powerful experience to be treated by different doctors who team up to put you back together. I know. I've been the guy lying on the field when the Giants' doctors and athletic trainers have come out to make sure that my knee or my hip isn't seriously injured. Then I make it to the sidelines and the medical staff continue to evaluate and treat me so I can get back on the playing field as soon as possible.

That's the way the New York Giants sports medicine team works, like a team. I know that's not always how it works in pro sports. You've got doctors and therapists and athletic trainers with a lot of degrees and a lot of knowledge among them, and the experts protect their turf. But on the Giants staff, they understand how to work together to give the players the best advice and best treatment. There's no ego involved. Dr. Kelly is an associate team doctor for the NY Giants and one of the top hip specialists in the country, but he's a personable guy. He's always been there to give me the right advice on treatment. Or he'll work with the other medical staff and team athletic trainers to come up with stretching or strengthening exercises for me.

When Dr. Rob came to the Giants, I'd been in the league for ten years. I had a lot of preexisting conditions, and I just thought, they're healed as well as they are going to heal. I was just going to have to live with the scar tissue and the restrictions, play as long as I could with it. But with Dr. Rob working on me, I got a new lease on life for the last part of my career. He's worked on everything from my neck to my shoulders to my back to my hips to my knees to my ankles to my feet to my toes! He's got rid of the restrictions, brought blood flow to these areas, and been involved in my rehab from surgery.

It's funny, you can tell in the locker room when someone is really effective. When Rob first came to the Giants, mostly only the older guys, such as myself and wide receiver Amani Toomer, used him. But last year, we're rushing to get to him before a game, because now it's freakin' crowded in the treatment room. All the younger guys are using him. Which lets you know the players believe in what he's doing.

The one game where everything came together, all the treatment and preparation, was the last game of my career, the 2008 Super Bowl. Now, by the end of the season, you're basically holding your body together with duct tape. But I made sure I worked with Rob every day of the two weeks leading up to the game—it was the big one and I wanted to get it right. When I went out there against the New England Patriots, it was the best I'd probably felt in ten years. I was leaping over people like a young guy again. One sack has become kind of famous, where my body is just hurtling horizontally at New England Patriots quarterback Tom Brady. I told Rob I could never have made that play without him and his muscle work. And I had confidence knowing that if I did get seriously hurt, Dr. Kelly had my back, or my hip.

It was the most amazing thing. I said to myself, "If I could have that much time to work on my muscles between every game, I could play forever." But I think all people at some point in their lives realize that their body is their business and that they had better take care of it. This book, *Muscle Medicine,* by two people who kept me in one piece, Bryan Kelly and Rob DeStefano, is the place you should start.

—Michael Strahan,
All-Pro New York Giants defensive end,
FOX Sports NFL studio analyst

1

INTRODUCING "MUSCLE MEDICINE"

We serve on the medical staff of the New York Giants and treat athletes at all skill levels, so it's fair to say we know something about the punishment the human body can take and dish out. But in our private practices, too much of the pain and suffering we see in our patients has no rationale whatsoever. It stems from a big and preventable cause: muscles are overlooked as an important piece of the treatment puzzle. A sore shoulder, a tight lower back, an achy knee— in virtually everyone over the age of thirty, these problems are so common, they're taken for granted as the near inevitable consequence of getting older. But that's just not true. Whether tight or injured muscle is the primary cause of pain and restriction or whether the main culprit is inside the joints, the tools exist to get to the root of the problem.

In the pages that follow, you will learn advanced muscle self-treatment techniques as well as stretching and strength exercises, all pegged to the most common body breakdowns. Merging our expertise as an orthopedic surgeon working in academic medicine and a sports chiropractor specializing in "hands-on" muscle therapies, we'll also show you how we treat more serious muscle and joint problems. Our aim is to put the tools of "muscle medicine" in your hands in the service of a pain-free life.

That our own backgrounds are so different has helped us appreciate how all the parts fit together. One of us, Dr. Bryan Kelly, is an orthopedic surgeon at the nation's premier orthopedic hospital, Manhattan's Hospital for Special Surgery, specializing in sports injuries to the hip, knee, and shoulder. He is also an assistant professor at Weill Cornell Medical College and is involved in a wide variety of research in sports medicine. The other of us, Dr. Robert DeStefano, was trained in chiropractic and, while developing busy practices in New Jersey and Manhattan, expanded his approach by teaching and developing hands-on muscle therapies. We have collaborated on both clinical and research protocols to improve the treatment strategies for patients with sports injuries.

What's different about our approach from others you may come across is that we look at the body the way nature made it, as an integrated system of bone, joint, and muscle. When there is pain or restriction, our job is to tease out the relationship among these three elements, so we can accurately diagnose and treat a musculoskeletal problem and, whenever possible, teach you how to treat yourself.

That doesn't *sound* radical, does it? But as the medical establishment evolved, different parts of the body became the territory of different specialists. Physical therapists work on muscle conditioning, trauma surgeons set bones and save lives, and sports medicine orthopedists repair joints. They all do valuable work, but what sometimes gets lost is an appreciation for how the whole system—bones, joints, and muscles—must be brought back into sync when everyday wear and tear knocks it out of kilter. (When we discuss specific injuries, you'll see how nerves can also interact with all three of these elements to contribute to pain and dysfunction.)

● **Dr. Kelly**

What do you do when you go to an orthopedic surgeon and he says there's no structural problem, nothing to fix? We say, there may be nothing wrong with you from his perspective, but it doesn't mean there's nothing wrong with you. It just means you can't see it on an MRI or X-ray. In this case the problem may be mostly muscular.

WHERE ARE THE MUSCLE DOCTORS?

In our experience, the approximately six hundred muscles in the body that keep humans upright and moving are often the most overlooked element of the system. Muscle is soft tissue that can't hold a surgeon's stitch—it basically heals itself—so it doesn't have its own branch of medical specialists to diagnose and treat it. Sure, any doctor will tell you muscles play a role in pain and dysfunction, but typically a supporting role—the stars of the show are supposed to be the joints, cartilage, and ligaments, in other words, the structures that show up damaged on an MRI. Minor muscle damage that may be seen on an MRI is often overlooked or viewed as clinically irrelevant. In addition, it's subjective—we don't yet have a numerical scale that measures muscle tightness. Yet experience has shown us that tight, damaged muscle can often be the primary cause of your problems. Even when muscle damage is the result of joint injury, it's often the factor that holds you back from complete recovery.

Take the example of a patient we treated not long ago. A former college soccer player turned business executive, he blew out the ACL (anterior cruciate ligament) in his knee playing club soccer. The surgery Dr. Kelly performed was a textbook reconstruction of the ligament, which restored stability to the knee joint. This patient seemed to have everything going for him—he was young, fit, and motivated—and yet after months of postsurgical physical therapy, he could still barely lift his leg. Dr. Kelly sent him to Dr. DeStefano, who broke up some scar tissue that had built up around the surgical site and lengthened the muscles that had tightened up after being immobilized postsurgery.

Our soccer player went back to physical therapy to strengthen the muscles and was running in weeks. The point is not that something is wrong with surgery or with physical therapy (both were absolutely necessary in this case) or magical about manual muscle therapy. The point is, the body returns to health in a sequence. First, tight or inflamed or scarred-down muscles have to heal before they can be conditioned to become stronger and more flexible. Exercise an injured muscle, even in a physical therapy setting, and it might not respond and you may just injure it some more.

INSIDE *MUSCLE MEDICINE*

Your musculoskeletal system takes a beating, whether from big traumas such as a torn ACL or simply from muscle and connective tissue in the joints growing inflexible and weaker with age. But some of the decline that is often written off as "normal aging" has less to do with the built-in deterioration of the cells themselves than with an accumulation of treatable muscular dinks and tweaks that were never addressed. Maybe your knees are achy and you can't jog or play basketball the way you used to, or your wrist is sore from working at the computer all day. Over time even the "small stuff" has a way of adding up to permanent pain, a lost range of motion, and a less active life. Which is not a small thing at all. In this book, we will briefly explain how the musculoskeletal system works, and sometimes falls apart, how the lifestyle choices you make affect the system, and ultimately, what you can do to recognize problems and often fix them yourself.

The *Muscle Medicine* approach to musculoskeletal health begins with a two-chapter look at the biology of muscles, joints, and bones, and at the events and forces that can do them harm. In Part Two, we move on to the choices you make in your everyday life that affect the system. A lot affects your body that's out of your hands, such as genetics (do both of your parents have surgically replaced hips?) and luck (did you suffer a serious knee injury playing high school sports?). In these chapters, we target three important areas where you can exert some control.

In chapter 4, "Mind-Body," you'll learn how psychological stress can wreak havoc on the mus-

● Dr. Kelly

It happens all the time. The patient comes in needing joint surgery, but their muscles are so weak, they can't lift their leg off the bed. I tell them, if we do surgery now, it's going to be a disaster. I send them to Rob for "prehab" to decrease the pain and improve the function of the muscles. Other patients don't necessarily need that, but if, after surgery, their muscles are shutting down or they've got a buildup of scar tissue, I send them for manual therapy on the muscles and it turns their rehab around. Now it's almost routine. Two or three months out from surgery, if I have any inkling at all that the muscles are getting into trouble or I want them better faster, I'll send patients for hands-on therapy. The muscle is ultimately what gets people back to normal. If you treat the bone and the joint and the muscle isn't functioning well, the patient is just not there.

culoskeletal system and how you can contain the damage by developing a measure of control over your thoughts and emotions. In chapter 5, "Nutrition," you'll learn how smart food choices can support bone growth and possibly reduce joint inflammation. We'll explain why maintaining a healthy weight will lessen the physical stress that wears down the joints. You get moving in chapter 6, with an all-around fitness plan that develops muscle and bone strength and cardio endurance, reducing the odds of injury.

In Part Three, we tour the body's seven "hot spots": neck; shoulder; elbow/ wrist/hand; lower back; hip; knee; ankle/foot. We focus on the most common sources of pain and the decisions that people make, or don't make, about how to deal with it. Do you ignore it? Do you stop running or swimming or playing your favorite sport? Do you explore self-treatment or seek out treatment from a muscle therapist, a physical therapist, an orthopedist? Not to be too dramatic about it, but by the time you hit your sixties, the answers to some of these questions could determine whether you're getting ready for tennis season or another physical therapy session.

In each hot spot, we'll describe the most common problems, how Dr. De-Stefano frees up tight and scarred-down tissues with "hands-on" manual techniques, and how, when the joint is seriously damaged, Dr. Kelly provides the orthopedic expertise. At the end of each of these chapters, you'll learn how to work on yourself, to protect against injury or to come back from it. We describe a series of self-treatment techniques tailored to each of the body's hot spots, based on the principles of Dr. DeStefano's muscle therapy. Using your hands and a few simple items such as a treatment stick and a physio ball, you'll learn to work directly on painfully contracted muscles to release the tissue and speed healing. Only when the area is no longer sore or inflamed will you progress to hot-spot-specific stretches to develop or maintain a healthy range of motion, and then strength exercises to build up resilience and protect against reinjury.

As you'll see, this book isn't a laundry list or an encyclopedia of musculoskeletal injuries. (If you're interested, plenty of books out there will give you the details of orthopedic procedures.) We've organized our information the same way we've taught ourselves to diagnose and treat problems, into three categories: Mostly Muscular; Muscle or Joint?; and Joint/Orthopedic. In the first group, which includes most problems, most of the time, injured muscle is generating the pain; any joint damage that shows up on an X-ray or an MRI is incidental. The standard medical prescription for this group is rest and a couple of Advil. Our approach is to get at the underlying causes and then to lay out a program to treat and strengthen all the important muscles in the hot spot.

With the problems that fall into our second category, Muscle or Joint?, neither the muscles nor the joint are working the way they're supposed to, and it's not clear who the most important bad actor is. Is the torn meniscus cartilage inside the knee the real issue, or can we bring the patient back to health just by working on the muscles that stabilize the joint? By putting these problems under a diagnostic microscope and always treating conservatively first, our goal is to eliminate avoidable surgeries.

Patients in the third group, Joint/Orthopedic, have serious damage inside the joint that must be addressed, medically or surgically. Here, we work on the muscles before (prehab) and after surgery (rehab) to shorten recovery times and improve the outcome. Mostly Muscular, Muscle or Joint?, Joint/Orthopedic—this isn't the standard approach to musculoskeletal injury, but in time we hope it will be.

The good news about these injuries is that the necessary expertise is out there to fix them, even if it's rarely collected under one roof—orthopedics to diagnose and repair joints; hands-on muscle therapy to promote muscle healing; and physical therapy/training to build up muscle and joint strength and flexibility. It's the team approach. Working with the New York Giants for the past six years, we've seen the results when players have access to the best talent from these different schools of treatment. We believe readers should have access to the same expertise, even if they're not (we hope) taking the same physical pounding as the Giants players.

FIGHTING BACK

Wouldn't it be nice if all-around healthy living were all that was needed to ward off muscle and joint problems? But no matter how you live your life, it's a near certainty that sooner or later you'll have to deal with musculoskeletal ills—they account for almost a quarter of the visits to primary-care physicians in this country. Young people playing competitive sports put their frames under tremendous pressure, from contact-sports body blows to the grinding repetition in the endurance-sports world. Adults find themselves in office jobs that have become hothouses for nagging aches and pains: lower-back pain from sitting glued to a desk; sore necks from improperly positioned computer screens; and overuse syndromes of the forearm—commonly if not always accurately labeled carpal tunnel syndrome—from all that typing and "mouse" wielding.

The lowest blow of all is that aging recreational athletes who maintain their cardiovascular fitness on the running trail, the tennis court, or in the gym are probably more susceptible to musculoskeletal damage than their couch-potato counterparts. (Ever notice how many social gatherings and dinner parties turn into a litany of "war wounds"?)

Muscle Medicine is a manual about fighting back: how to make the right choices to address both healthy and damaged muscle, whether it's on your own or with professional care. It lays out the first truly integrative approach to the care and repair of muscle and joint problems. Whether you're an accomplished athlete, you want to maintain your regular tennis routine, or you just want to be able to play with your kids, or your grandkids, without back pain after a long day at the office, we want to be on your team.

● Dr. DeStefano

Every day, I treat patients who are convinced that the source of their pain is the damage inside their joint that shows up on an X-ray or MRI. A patient will come in and say, "Can you help me with my meniscus tear in my knee?" I'll say, "No, I can't help you with the meniscus tear, but I may be able to help you with the pain in your knee." What people don't usually understand is that in many cases, if we can get the muscles around the joint to move properly, the joint itself doesn't have to be in perfect shape for the system to work without pain. That's something I can appreciate. I've been in two serious accidents—once when a car hit me while I was training for the Ironman World Championships and once in a Manhattan cab crash—and I've got the chipped vertebrae and herniated disks to show for it. A year ago, the pain in my back and neck flared up so badly, my orthopedist was ready to bring in a neurosurgeon to work me up for disk surgery. I kept exercising, getting manual therapy, and applying self-treatment. Slowly, over a month, the contracted muscles in my cervical and lumbar spine let go their grip, and the pain went away. I'm not cured; I still have damaged disks. I may need surgery down the line, but as long as I'm symptom-free and maintain the health of my muscles, I'm fine.

PART

1

These next two chapters will introduce you to the biology of your musculo-skeletal system. In chapter 2, "How the System Works," you'll learn about the basic building blocks of the system—muscles, bones, and joints. In chapter 3, "System Malfunction," you'll be exposed to the major forces, internal and external, that can tear the system down.

YOUR BODY

HOW THE SYSTEM WORKS:
MUSCLES, BONES, JOINTS

Before we talk about lifestyle issues or jump into the nuts and bolts of body problems, let's first admire the machinery and come to a basic understanding of how it works. As we've said, muscles and bones and joints form one integrated system, and no one component is more important than another. Without muscles, you would be a motionless pile of bones; without a skeleton, you'd look and move more like a jellyfish; and without joints to control and stabilize the bones, you'd stumble around like the scarecrow from the *Wizard of Oz*.

MUSCLES

The muscles under your conscious control—skeletal muscles—are the motors that drive the human system. (The smooth muscle that lines the organs and the cardiac muscle that keeps your heart beating are involuntary.) The muscles function in tandem. As one muscle shortens it exerts a pulling force, while at the same time its counterpart relaxes. This simultaneous action of a contracting *agonist* muscle and a relaxing *antagonist* muscle powers all the movements of the body. That's the case whether it's a sprinter thrusting his lead leg forward (the massive quadriceps muscles in the front of the thigh contracting, the hamstrings in back relaxing) or you bending your finger to scratch your nose (flexor digitorum contracts, extensor digitorum relaxes).

Controlling the movements of so many muscles is precision work that is initiated and coordinated in the brain. The process might seem as simple as turning on a light switch, but in reality, it's a constant neurochemical conversation between the nerves and the muscles. That is, the brain oversees the production of specific chemicals that activate the muscles. What happens is this: the brain sends a chemical message to the motor neurons in the spinal cord which then deliver that message to the target muscle, telling it what to do. Sensory nerves gather information about the current status of that part of the body and send that information back up the spinal cord to the brain for processing. Some information is so basic, it doesn't need to be processed by the brain: it travels only from the muscles to the spinal cord and back, in a feedback loop called a "reflex arc." For example, the muscles have reflexes that prevent them from overstretching or overcontracting, or that jerk your hand off a hot stove before you even register pain.

A more complex conversation between the muscles, nerves, and brain is called "proprioception"—knowing where your body is in space. It allows you to run and jump and navigate the world without falling (usually) or even thinking much about it. When you're injured, that conversation is disrupted. Not only do the muscle tissues have to heal, but the lines of communication between the muscle and the brain have to be reestablished so you can run or swing a golf club or play a note on the violin with your brain on "automatic pilot."

But it's how muscles interact with each other and the rest of the body that most concerns us here. Muscle is dense with capillaries that feed it with the blood—carrying oxygen and nutrients—that it needs to do its work. We may think of the football player with big muscles as rugged and tough, but the muscle tissue itself is surprisingly delicate, made up mostly of water. (They don't call it soft tissue for nothing.) The body is closely packed with overlapping muscles that must move smoothly against each other if humans are to move with any fluidity.

From micro to macro, the master plan is steady, unimpeded motion—movement is life. Not only do neighboring muscles need to slide against each other, so do the fiber bundles inside the individual muscles, and so again, the tiny myofibrils inside the fibers. We can see what muscular contraction looks like at the most basic molecular level only with an electron microscope: two types of protein filaments inside the myofibrils, actin and myosin, pulling against each other.

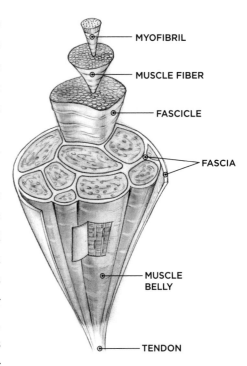

The defining aspect of the muscle is the muscle "belly," where most of the muscular force is generated. Fortunately, nature has outfitted the muscle with tough connective tissue at both ends, the tendons, where the muscle attaches to the bone. The tendons transmit muscular force and actually pull on the bones. Remember, regular muscle tissue can't even hold a surgeon's stitch, much less control a bone in motion. (Our word *muscle* comes from the Latin word for mouse, *mus*. The cord- or band-shaped tendons were thought to resemble the snout and the tail of a mouse!)

Another element of the muscle package is the fascia, the thin, tough, translucent membrane that weaves around everything in the body: muscles, bones, organs, nerves, the works. You could visualize it as the casing around the meat in a string of sausages. Or take a close look at an uncooked chicken or slab of beef. It's the white covering around the muscle that runs through it and around it. In the body (human, cow, or chicken), fascia serves as a kind of flexible internal skeleton, holding the muscles in place, but also moving with them, and helping them slide over neighboring structures.

BONES

You take for granted that your muscles are a living, dynamic system. Work out in the gym even for just a few weeks and you'll see the strength and, depending on the amount of testosterone circulating in your system, the size of your muscles increase. (Inside the muscles, the numbers of capillaries increase, pumping up the fluid content; new protein—the building block of muscle—is laid down; the mitochondria—the power plants inside the cells—increase in density.)

The skeleton might seem rather inert, by comparison, a convenient frame to which muscles and organs are attached. True, after you stop growing in your teens or early twenties, your bones don't get any longer. But your skeleton is a system as alive as any other in the body. About a third of bone is made up of living cells. Inside the bone, marrow cells are producing red and white blood cells, as well as other cells that help drive the immune system.

The outside of the bone is covered by a fibrous membrane, the periosteum, which contains blood vessels and nerves. (When you break a bone, it's the ruptured periosteum that causes the pain.) But even the two-thirds of the bone made up of hard mineral (mostly calcium phosphate) isn't static. Bone is always slowly but constantly being reshaped. Special cells called osteoclasts eat away at old or damaged bone. This activity is balanced by that of the osteoblast cells, which create new bone. Bone is reabsorbed where it is not needed and laid down where it is. As overall bone density drops significantly in the senior years (those osteoclasts gain the upper hand in the end), it's up to you to stress the system in healthful ways (i.e., activate the osteoblasts by lifting weights, or walking) so that it stays resilient enough to handle the bumps of everyday life. In other words, use it or lose it.

JOINTS

Movement happens when muscles generate the force to move the bones. But we need a third component, a simple mechanism that allows bones to articulate, to move against each other, so that actual work—lifting, lowering, etc.—can occur. We call these mechanisms joints. Let's take the simple action of lifting your forearm. The top end of the biceps muscle attaches in the shoulder area; this is the muscle's *origin,* its stable, anchoring point. The other end of the muscle attaches to the moving bone at the *insertion,* in this case, just below the elbow joint. Anchored at the shoulder, the biceps muscle contracts, lifting up the forearm. The biceps is the agonist muscle, and when it fires, the antagonist muscle, the triceps, releases. A muscle can only pull as it contracts. It's got no "push" mode, which is why muscles have to work together. When it's time for that forearm to lower, the triceps, now the agonist, contracts, and the biceps, now the antagonist, relaxes, and the deed is done.

Most of the joints we'll be talking about in this book function as lever systems. In other words, the joint translates the individual efforts of a number of muscles into a decisive, coordinated movement of the limbs. The knee and the elbow are hinges that only allow movement in one or two directions; the ankle and the wrist allow more freedom of movement. The hip and the shoulder are ball-in-socket joints with the greatest range. Every joint makes its own trade-off between strength, stability, and range of motion.

The joint's purpose is to provide the bones with the maximum movement, the necessary stability, and a minimum of friction. The bones that form the joint fit into a sleeve called a joint capsule, which is filled with lubricating synovial fluid. The ends of the bones inside the capsule are covered with smooth articular cartilage that allows them to move against each other without grinding. Finally, outside the joint, synovial-fluid-filled sacs called bursas provide an extra measure of musculo-skeletal cushioning.

The tough outer layer of the joint capsule is made from another kind of carti-lage, fibrocartilage. Some joints have special fibrocartilage shock absorbers inside the capsule—the labrum in the shoulder and hip, and the meniscus in the knee. In the spine, fibrocartilage makes up the disks, filled with mucoprotein gel, that act as shock absorbers between the vertebrae.

Inside, and sometimes outside, the capsule, strong bands of tissue called liga-ments connect the two bones together and hold them in place, allowing for con-trolled movement. (The ligaments in the knee are the most numerous and also the most often torn.) The common denominator for all these structures, what really makes the system work, is collagen: a tough, rubbery, and altogether amazing ma-terial that is the building block of all the connective tissues in the body—cartilage and ligament, as well as muscular fascia and tendon.

No question, the joints are impressively engineered; the detail can be mind-boggling. But it's worth remembering that the muscles are very effective shock absorbers, possibly absorbing up to—or more than—half the force you generate, whether you're eluding tacklers on the football field or sitting at the desk. Between the muscles and the joints, it might seem as if nature had devised a bulletproof system for moving around in the world, barring a car accident or a severe sports injury, impervious to breakdown. If you're over thirty-five or forty, you know that's not true. We'll take up that story in the next chapter.

SYSTEM MALFUNCTION:
WHEN THINGS BREAK DOWN

If you want to hold someone or something accountable for muscle and joint problems that pile up as people age, blame evolution. A couple of million years ago, our animal ancestors changed from walking on all fours to standing tall on two, but the human musculoskeletal system has never really fully adapted. The adult human head is a real cannonball, weighing eight to twelve pounds. If you have poor posture, that weight can contribute to problems in the neck area. The entire trunk weighs down on the lower back. Our frames still haven't made their peace with gravity.

Age really exposes the design flaws. If you have the good fortune to escape joint injury when you're young, the middle and senior years are when you're most likely to bump against the shelf life of the materials you're made out of. (This wasn't such an issue for most of human history when the average life span was a fraction of what it is today.)

BONES

Let's go back to the three basic components of the human frame: bones, joints, and muscles. Owing to its mostly mineral composition, bone is fairly rigid and, not surprisingly, fractures if it's subjected to sufficient impact. But bone is living material. With the exception of broken bones in seniors (or smokers or anyone else with low bone density), a fracture stimulates the bone-building osteoblast cells to patch up the break so completely, it heals stronger than new. Men's skeletons rarely slow them down until well into their senior years, when the osteoclasts, the "breaking-down" cells, leach so much mineral out of the bones, they become vulnerable to fracture. In the most common scenario, the bony vertebrae of the back suffer microfractures, causing the spinal column to compress, taking off a few inches of height. In women, bone health, like so many other things, is influenced by the sex hormones. When estrogen levels drop off dramatically during meno-pause, women are vulnerable to dangerous bone thinning or osteoporosis. For se-nior women, a fractured hip is a potentially life-threatening injury. (We'll talk about ways to protect bone density with diet and exercise in chapters 5 and 6.)

JOINTS

The joints have a tough job. They must stabilize the bones as they move inside the joint capsule, and they bear the heaviest responsibility for supporting the weight of the body. The routine act of climbing or walking down stairs places on the knee a load equal to three or four times your body weight. As we described in the previ-ous chapter, the joints can handle these forces thanks to connective tissue that runs in and around them—tendons, ligaments, and cartilage—all composed mostly of collagen. Collagen's spongy, matrixlike structure permits these connective tissues to compress and expand, responding to the forces placed on them with just the right balance of firmness and flexibility.

Some joint trauma is so severe, it makes no difference how young and lithe you are. Twist your knee a certain way as your skis slide out from under you and you'll tear your ACL. But as you age, your connective tissue loses water and becomes less supple, making you more vulnerable to injury from the accumulation of every-day stresses and strains. The two most common examples of this are probably the injuries to the disks in your lower back and the meniscus cartilage in your knee. Both are shock-absorbing structures made of fibrocartilage that dries out over time. When the tissues deteriorate, it doesn't take much—a single awkward twist, and you've cracked (or "herniated") a disk, or torn that flat, C-shaped meniscus inside the knee. If you're over forty and you've escaped this fate, you probably have at least one or two friends who haven't.

Injuries to the structures inside a joint are almost always serious because the tissue there heals so poorly, or not at all. The orthopedic surgeon steps in where nature can't. If you tear your ACL, you do without or you get it surgically repaired. It's a case-by-case proposition. Some knee ligament and meniscus tears will heal, slowly, but only in young patients. (The robust circulation of youth pumps up the otherwise modest blood supply to these areas.) The tendons, the connective tissues that attach muscle to bone, are also slow healers. In the case of severe tendon tears, the surgeon surgically repairs them to bone.

But the mother of all nonhealers is the articular cartilage, the tissue that cushions the ends of the bones inside the joint. Inside the joint capsule, there is no blood supply—the cartilage is nourished by the synovial fluid. When the cartilage sustains damage from trauma at any age, or from wear and tear as it gets older and drier, it has minimal or no ability to heal itself. No joint is immune from nicks and scratches over time. But in the larger joints such as the hip, the knee, and the shoulder, the damage can cross a threshold and become self-perpetuating. As the cartilage thins, the bones inside the joint capsule begin to move abnormally, further injuring the cartilage and setting off the body's inflammatory response. Eventually, the cartilage can completely disappear, until bone is rubbing against bone, producing pain, restriction of movement, and injury to the bone tissue itself. This is very bad news for the joints as it can result in osteoarthritis. (Rheumatoid arthritis is a different beast. Not as common as osteoarthritis, it's an autoimmune disease in which the body's own defenses attack the joints, usually smaller, finer ones such as the fingers and wrists.)

It's a grim-sounding scenario. But the important thing to remember is that even though genetics and injury can play their part, the choices you make may determine whether you cross the finish line with your original joints intact. Low-impact movement is your friend, a sedentary lifestyle is not. (We'll discuss this in more detail in chapter 6 and in the individual "Hot Spots" chapters.)

MUSCLES

Let's turn our attention to the muscles that power all that useful movement. If joints are, sometimes, the weak links in the musculoskeletal system, the muscles that drive them are their most resilient defenders. They absorb much of the physical force to which the body is subjected. (Recall the jolt your knee took when you didn't see the curb coming and your foot smacked down on the road surface before your leg muscles had the chance to flex and cushion the shock.) When the muscles are firing strongly, they can compensate for a joint whose internal moving parts are not at the peak of health. Here's a dramatic example. Not long ago, we treated a talented recreational marathoner. In his last race, everything had been going according to plan until late in the race when he'd been shut down by hip pain. We were floored when his X-rays revealed he had advanced osteoarthritis in his hip. His trained athlete's muscles were functioning at such a high level, he was running marathons when a sedentary person with the same degree of the disease would have spent the past five years hobbling in pain. Of course, our marathoner is an extreme case and a cautionary tale as well. (A hip replacement and the end of his running career were in his near future.) Your goal is to have healthy muscles that support healthy (or healthy enough) joints.

We know from the research literature that joint damage by itself is often not the whole story behind pain and restriction. In a famous 1994 study published in the *New England Journal of Medicine,* 64 percent of the subjects, none of whom suffered from back pain, had significant disk abnormalities that turned up on their MRI exams. Similar studies have looked at meniscus tears in the knee, which, according to one Harvard paper, are found in one out of three people over the age of forty-five, only a fraction of which cause symptoms.

Now let's look at muscle fiber. Like connective tissue, muscle ages over time, losing water and suppleness and becoming more vulnerable to injury. Unlike bone, which usually heals better than new, muscle tears heal themselves with a second-rate patch material: scar tissue made from collagen that is stiffer and weaker than the original fibers. But in contrast to connective tissue, muscle has a great blood supply. It's packed with capillaries that bring in oxygen and nutrients, allowing the tissue to heal quickly (if imperfectly), and the healthy muscles can grow bigger and stronger in response to healthy stress.

If no effort is made, muscle mass and muscle endurance will decline about 1 percent a year after the age of forty. All of the body's systems decline with age, but nothing bounces back like muscle responding to exercise. In one famous study by a University of Arkansas researcher, some hundred-year-old study subjects doubled their strength with a program of light weight training. (Certainly, American swimmer Dara Torres has opened a few eyes, defeating competitors less than half her age with her three silver medals at the Beijing Olympics.) Muscle is the human equivalent of a renewable power resource like wind or solar energy. Connective tissue, especially articular cartilage, is more like oil, nonrenewable. When it starts to run out, you scramble to adapt, and when it's gone, it's gone.

To power the body and protect the joints, muscles have to respond to a command from the nervous system with a simultaneous contraction and relaxation of the agonist and the antagonist. When they can't, its often the result of muscle dysfunction or injury, the two major categories being traumatic and chronic injury. In the case of trauma, the damage is the work of a moment: a trip, a fall, a car accident. The most common example of muscle trauma is a strain—or a "pulled" muscle—when the muscles fibers overstretch and tear. How many tear determines the severity of the strain. (As a matter of terminology, muscles suffer *strains,* and ligaments, when they are stretched and ripped, suffer *sprains.*) In the simplest cases, a muscle is asked to contract too hard or for too long, and something "gives," for instance when an out-of-shape recreational athlete decides to start the season with wind sprints and pulls a hamstring muscle.

TRAUMATIC VS. CHRONIC MUSCLE INJURY

But what if the muscle pull isn't a one-shot deal? Let's say you keep suffering muscle pulls in the same place. Or the joint and the surrounding muscle get achier and weaker from the stress of everyday life. Now we've entered the realm of chronic injury. Something has gone awry in the way the muscles and the joints work together that produces constant irritation. The most common forms of chronic trouble are labeled repetitive stress injuries. Think about performing the same small, rapid movement over and over without giving the muscles a chance to rest and recover, for example, clicking a computer mouse all day. Little tears develop in the muscles and the connective tissue; the area becomes inflamed and then chronically sore. These

FIVE REASONS MUSCLES ARE WEAK

1. **Underuse:** This may cause pain and dysfunction, possibly affecting other muscles and joints along the "kinetic chain." A good example would be the gluteal muscles in the butt, which aren't used much by distance runners. Their weakness causes the hips to move laterally during running and may add to muscular imbalances, an inefficient stride, and the possibility of lower-leg injuries.
2. **Fatigue from overwork:** Muscles may tire out trying to stabilize an unstable structure. When you sit for long periods, the muscles of the lumbar spine can become weak or tired and painfully tight, fighting a losing battle against gravity and poor posture.
3. **Nerve damage:** If a nerve going to a muscle is damaged, the muscle can't properly fire. Despite the tissue's potential, the body can't communicate with it, so the muscle will test as weak. And if the nerve problem isn't corrected, over time the muscle will atrophy from lack of use.
4. **Infection:** The muscle is using its resources to fight the infection. In this condition, it will test as a weak muscle.
5. **Muscle disease:** A disease such as muscular dystrophy will cause progressive muscle weakness and atrophy.

repetitive stress injuries have become the bane of the workplace, and are increasingly considered the most common form of occupational injury, costing the nation, by some estimates, more than $100 billion a year in medical costs, decreased productivity, and other related expenses. The two biggies that we'll discuss in the "Hot Spots" section are carpal tunnel syndrome and lower-back pain. Interestingly, in the latter case, the problem isn't too much movement but too little. The postural muscles have to work so hard to keep the spine aligned when the body is sitting in a fixed position that they tire out and become irritated.

The line between traumatic and chronic injury is anything but hard and fast. Sometimes a muscle trauma can destabilize a joint area, setting it up for chronic problems. Sometimes chronic inflammation can weaken the muscles or connective tissue to such a degree that an otherwise ordinary pivot or twist can cause structures to rip—the straw that broke the camel's back. But let's go beyond standard textbook terms and take a closer look at the different ways muscle can cause pain and limit movement before we consider the ways to treat it.

When muscle is asked to do too much, to fire too long or too hard, it can simply tighten up and shut down in self-defense so forcefully as to cause pain. But the tricky thing about diagnosing muscle pain is that the site of the original tissue damage is sometimes not where it hurts the most. This is one reason muscle problems can be mistaken for joint injury. Muscle can refer pain to other areas of the body in several ways. Sometimes a contracted muscle will press down on a nerve sending pain (or numbness or tingling) to some other part of the body along that nerve track; for instance, a compressed sciatic nerve in the back can cause pain down the leg. Sometimes an overwhelmed muscle just shuts down, forcing neighboring muscles to pick up the slack, and then *they* become fatigued and painful. Restriction in one part of the muscle can pull on the tendon where it attaches the muscle to the bone, causing pain there. Diagnosis in these cases of "referred pain" can be tricky, and the bigger musculoskeletal picture needs to be considered. Just because you have pain in the lower back doesn't mean that is the source of the problem and the location that needs to be treated first. This is why it is so important to see a doctor and not try to self-diagnose!

The tendon is a popular area for pain. Everyone has heard of tendinitis, the inflammation that sets in when tendons and the surrounding muscle are overstressed and overstretched. "Tennis elbow" (lateral epicondylitis) and Achilles tendinitis are all-too-common examples. But in fact, the latest research is telling us that the tendons have only a limited capacity to become inflamed. Chronic pain is usually produced by the deterioration of the tendon's collagen fibers, a downward spiral of microscopic tearing and scarring better described by the term *tendonosis*. Conventional medicine has had only limited success treating tendonosis with anti-inflammatory drugs. And it doesn't pay much attention to the potential root cause of the problem: overly contracted muscle fibers that pull on the tendon ends.

Finally, in the case of a serious joint injury, muscle problems are not the cause, but the effect. Pain receptors inside the joint detect something disturbing about the way the joint is moving, and they send signals to the muscles telling the joint to slow or shut down, minimizing the chance of further damage. You see this "guarding reflex" in nature all the time such as when an animal limps with a leg drawn up so as not to further stress an injured joint. Humans, of course, are good at over-

REFERRAL PATTERNS

Very often, the muscles refer pain to other parts of the body. In other words, the symptoms of an injured or irritated muscle can be felt in areas other than the actual damage site. This makes diagnosis and treatment difficult at times and can be very confusing for the patient. The following charts illustrate the most common muscle referral patterns. The shaded areas represent spots where you may feel all or just some of each muscle's referred pain.

1. Psoas [A]
2. Gluteus Maximus [C]
3. Piriformis [E]

4. Upper Trapezius [G]
5. Biceps [I]
6. Scalenes [K]

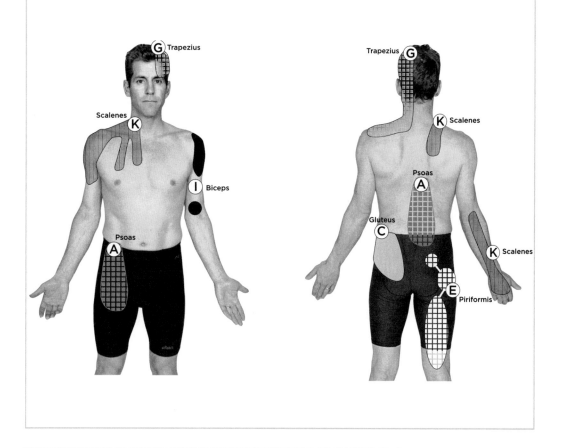

riding their body with their brain, choosing to finish their run or their basketball game even though their knee or hip is aching and the muscles around it have tightened up.

As we've seen, when damaged muscle is the primary problem, the immediate source of pain may be the nerves, the tendons, the muscle fibers themselves, or a combination of the three. Fortunately, hands-on muscle therapies have shown themselves to be effective at getting to the source of the problem: tight muscles.

When treating muscle, the manual therapist has to contend with the secondary damage brought about by inflammation. In the case of a traumatic injury, inflammation is a good thing, at first. It's the body's attempt to protect itself against further injury, and start the healing process, by flooding the area with plasma, fluid, and immune cells. But if the injured area remains irritated, or the problem is chronic, inflammation settles in for a longer stay and becomes part of the problem, not the solution. The muscle fibers remain locked in contraction, clamping down on the capillaries and reducing blood flow through the area. This has a doubly bad effect, reducing the supply of oxygen into the tissues and the flow of metabolic waste products out.

In this distressed environment, the body lays down collagen-based scar tissue to stabilize the area. In the case of an acute injury, this makes sense. It's the only patch material muscles have. But in a chronic situation, it just gums up the works. These microscopic adhesions impede the way the fibers inside the muscle move against each other, and the way the muscle slides over neighboring muscles and nerves, and how it moves within the broad layer of fascia that gives shape to the entire soft-tissue system. The friction creates more inflammation and swelling, triggering the formation of yet more adhesions, and so on.

HANDS-ON MUSCLE THERAPY

Manual therapy has more than one way to pull muscle tissue out of this downward spiral. Massage therapies have been around for centuries as all-purpose body tonics. Massage stimulates the circulatory system to bring blood back to oxygen-starved muscles and helps the lymphatic system flush out waste. Modern therapeutic schools such as Active Release Techniques (ART) and Trigger Point Therapy have brought manual therapy into the twenty-first century, drawing on scientific anatomy and physiology to target damaged muscles. They can trace their roots back to ancient China and the development of acupressure and then acupuncture therapies. (The creator of Trigger Point Therapy, a pioneering M.D. named Janet Travell, served as personal physician to both President John Kennedy and President Lyndon Johnson.)

It's beyond the scope of this book to offer a who's who of manual therapies. Dr. DeStefano, though well versed in a number of different muscle techniques, predominately uses ART. While that certainly influences the way we discuss the treatment of the various hot-spot issues, our emphasis is not on the specific treatment techniques, but on understanding and diagnosing problems that can be treated manually in a variety of ways. No scientific rationale for one form of manual therapy being "better" than another exists; some therapists have had excellent success combining therapies that have very different theoretical underpinnings, for instance, ART and acupuncture. Many ART practitioners, including Dr. DeStefano, believe in the value of combining muscle work with chiropractic treatments to address a range of musculoskeletal problems.

Over the past decade or so, researchers in academic physical therapy have filled in our understanding of the physiology of distressed muscles. But we still don't know how exactly the different schools of manual therapy get the good results that they do. Every manual therapy has its dogma, but unlike many medical and surgical treatments, there is not a lot of supporting hard science.

Exciting research *is* being published that looks at the key role fascia plays, binding together muscles, joints, and bones in a single interconnected system. Researchers are doing groundbreaking work on a class of molecular receptors called integrins. These molecules seem to permit the different cells of the musculoskeletal system to communicate, so that when, for example, the arm moves, everything from skin to bone moves as a coordinated whole.

In the coming years, this research may give us a better theoretical handle on what we're doing when we manually work on muscle or, for that matter, when we cut through muscle to surgically repair joints. But the focus of this book is mostly practical, helping to ensure that your muscles and joints work as well, and last as long, as the rest of you.

The next three chapters map out a program to build up the resilience of your musculoskeletal system, protecting it against injury and plain old everyday life. In chapter 4, "Mind-Body," you'll learn how psychological stress can wreak havoc on the system and how to contain the damage by developing a measure of control over your stress. In chapter 5, "Nutrition," you'll learn how smart food choices can build up the durability of the system by supporting bone growth and reducing inflammation in your joints. And by maintaining a healthy weight, you reduce the physical stress that wears the body down. In chapter 6, "Fitness," you get moving. Using our exercise principles and our favorite exercises, you'll build your own all-around "functional" fitness program that develops balance, cardio endurance, and muscle and bone strength, enhancing your health and cutting down the chance of injury.

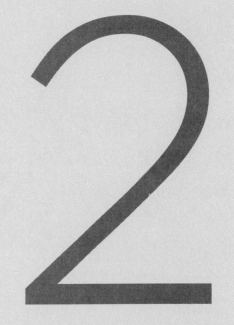

PART

2

RESILIENCE

MIND-BODY

We're paid to work on patients' muscles and joints, not their psyches. And we don't claim to understand the exact nature of the relationship between mind and body (who does?), but we can't help but observe how deep those connections are and how important they can be. Let's take breathing, for example. As you may recall from the last chapter, inflamed, contracted tissues reduce blood flow, and therefore the supply of oxygen, to an area,

> **Dr. DeStefano**
>
> There is a strong link between emotional stress and muscular dysfunction. It's not merely stress which causes physical problems. It's the expression of that stress and how it is stored and displayed as a physical manifestation, or rather, how that particular patient reacts to and handles that stress. Some may not show any physical symptoms at all, while another may store and physically manifest stress. Patients will sometimes burst into tears in my office. Sometimes it's from the stress of the pain while other times it's a result of emotional stress. A box of Kleenex in the office can come in very handy.

● Dr. Kelly

I believe the psychological state of a patient has a huge impact on recovery. Some of what I do during my office hours is positive reinforcement: "No, you're doing fine, it's supposed to hurt, you just had surgery." People get frustrated at the time it takes to recover from surgery. They'll say, "I went down to the beach and walked three miles and all of a sudden my hip started killing me. And I didn't do anything." I'll tell them, "Well, your hip thinks it's something. And it's normal for you to feel frustrated or depressed, but that's not helping your recovery. If you're optimistic and positive and feel good about things, you'll get better faster."

leading to the formation of microscopic scar tissue. That's what's going on at the micro level. At the macro level, well, let's say you're stressed-out at work or at home. Without being consciously aware of it, you respond by taking rapid, shallow breaths (which take in less oxygen) and by tensing up. The muscles in your lower back, neck and shoulders, and buttocks tighten into a hunched, defensive posture as if you're protecting yourself from life's blows. The consequence: less total oxygen passing through the lungs and even less reaching those restricted muscles.

"ILLNESS BEHAVIOR"

As we'll discuss in detail in the lumbar-spine hot-spot chapter, lower-back pain can be particularly excruciating. What is the sufferer's reasonable, but counterproductive, reaction? You rest in bed. (For an acute back spasm, some bed rest, but not much, could be helpful.) When you do emerge, you are careful to avoid the usual activities that work those back muscles—long walks, jogging, chores in or outside the house—for fear of triggering another disabling attack. In the walking you can't eliminate, you favor the side that hurts by putting more weight on the opposite leg. When you walk, you tilt.

This is an example of what experts sometimes call illness behavior. In other words, you do things to make yourself ill even though that's the last thing you would consciously choose. Restricting your activities weakens the muscles, making them less efficient shock absorbers. As the muscle fibers shorten and tighten, they become more prone to strain and pain. When you adjust your gait or the way you hold your shoulders to baby the painful area, you throw off the body's normal biomechanics and overstrain the compensating muscles. Try an experiment. Actually, don't try it, but imagine it—walk around for a day with a slightly bent-over, crooked posture, what's called an antalgic gait. By the end of the day, your lower back really will hurt and you won't be acting anymore.

Remember, movement is life. Your back may not be 100 percent. But a long walk or, if you're a runner, a slow jog might bring blood flow and oxygen to the area and could speed up healing.

Now we come to the mind part of the mind-body equation. If you've been lugging a heavy suitcase on vacation for a week and your lower back acts up, emotional soul-searching probably isn't necessary: don't indulge in illness behavior, get moving, and it will probably pass. But if back pain is your intermittent or chronic companion, then psychological issues may well be relevant whether or not, for instance, there is significant underlying damage to the spinal disks. Most obviously, the fear of crippling back spasms contributes to the muscle tension that generates, or at least contributes to, the pain—a vicious cycle. More subtly, a range of negative emotions may be bound up in trying to cope with that pain. While cause and effect are far from established, a hefty research literature has established that people who are depressed or who feel that they lack control in their lives are more likely to suffer from chronic pain. In one famous Stanford study, psychological test scores were a far better predictor of future back-pain problems than any structural damage that showed up on an X-ray or MRI.

THE MIND GAME

The person who has waged the most radical attack on the old conventional wisdom that damaged disks explain most intense back pain is a New York City doctor of rehabilitative medicine, John Sarno. Sarno's influence within the medical profession has been limited, but his 1991 bestseller, *Healing Back Pain,* has persuaded impressive numbers of readers that the source of their back troubles is in their head. Tight muscles and a restricted supply of oxygen causes the pain, he says, but that's only a physical mechanism triggered by repressed negative emotions, especially anger. The back or neck pain is an unconscious diversion strategy for people who would rather deal with their physical than their psychic pain. Confront the source of that psychic pain, he says, whatever it may be, and the physical problem will go away, usually sooner rather than later.

These days, even the most conservative orthopedic surgeons agree that emotional stress can play a role in back pain. They'll also point out that damaged disks do often contribute to the most serious back-pain cases. Whether we agree with Dr. Sarno's theory that the unconscious mind lurks behind every case of muscle-related back pain is another question, one that's outside the scope of this book. However, if we can look past the negative comments Dr. Sarno makes about his colleagues, we can agree with his basic concept: in many cases, if you relax, stop contracting tight muscles, and learn to deal with emotional stress, you can reduce or eliminate pain.

Although we agree that back pain can be a physical manifestation of repressed emotions, our treatment approach is our major area of difference with the doctor. No matter what first causes muscles to tighten up, once they remain locked in contraction, harmful physical changes take place, including oxygen starvation and scar-tissue formation. Much of this book is devoted to explaining and describing how manual therapies address those physical changes at a physical level. If, for instance, you're lucky enough not to have a "weak link" in your musculoskeletal system, you may just experience generalized muscle tension. But if you have a "bad back," or chronically tight neck muscles, that's the reactive area where stress is going to manifest. Unless you deal with those damaged muscles, stress may always gravitate there.

To us, a muscle medicine worthy of the name addresses both mind and body. When you're dealing with chronic back and neck pain, why not use all the tools available, the ones that get at the physical symptoms as well as the possible emotional underpinnings. So we coach patients on stress-reduction techniques. Whereas conventional psychological therapy gets patients to focus on their individual life issues, our stress-reduction exercises work to make people more aware of universal body processes such as breathing that have a big influence on their emotional life. Quieting fearful or angry emotions can lessen muscle tension and pain, and that's a good thing.

As with all forms of treatment, timing is essential. If you're having a lower-back spasm, you want a muscle therapist to help bring you out of pain before you give much thought to the emotions that may have triggered it. Likewise, if you're having a heart attack, you'd like medical science to save your life, then it may be time to contemplate stress management. (That's a dramatic example but not an idle one. Heart disease is the country's number one killer; stress is a leading cause of heart disease.)

STRESS AND STRESS REDUCTION

Before we move on to specific mind-body exercises, let's take a closer look at this thing, stress, that your mind and your body are up against. Stress is the body's response to being overwhelmed by the outside world. For much of human evolutionary history, the outside world was trying to kill us—predators, environmental exposure, you name it—so our species evolved a hormonal mechanism to jump-start us into taking life-saving action, the so-called fight-or-flight response. The brain orders the endocrine system to produce stress hormones such as adrenaline that pump up the heart rate and send our nervous system into high gear. That's great for fighting or fleeing tigers, but in the modern world, the threats to our well-being are more often psychological. Our stress response stays jammed in the "on" position without a satisfying physical release to turn it off. Most of the chronic diseases and disorders of the past century are either caused or made worse by this kind of unresolved hyperstress.

In the early 1970s, Western science began to look at the health benefits of breathing and meditation exercises, and their ability to turn off the stress hormones controlled by the sympathetic nervous system and turn on the counteracting parasympathetic nervous system. Pioneering Harvard researcher Herbert Benson documented the slowed-down heart and breathing rates of meditating subjects and dubbed this the relaxation response. Since the late seventies, an MIT-trained biologist, Jon Kabat-Zinn, has been using meditation techniques as the basis for an influential stress-reduction program at the University of Massachusetts Medical School at Worcester, generating research and helping people get a better handle on their emotional and physical problems, including chronic muscle pain. The program Kabat-Zinn founded, now called the Center for Mindfulness in Medicine, Health Care, and Society (www.umassmed.edu/cfm/index.aspx), and his first book, *Full Catastrophe Living: Using the Wisdom of Your Body and Mind to Face Stress, Pain, and Illness,* are excellent places to start digging deeper into the mind-body approach to muscle pain.

Drawing on Benson, Kabat-Zinn, and others, we've come up with a short list of stress-reduction exercises that over the years some of our patients have enjoyed and benefited from. The common thread is encouraging patients to slow down and become aware (or *mindful,* to use the term borrowed from the Buddhist meditation tradition) of just how frantic their lives really are. Keep in mind that stress can be good. It motivates us to get to work on time and get things done. Stress itself doesn't cause problems; it's the way we handle it that's the issue. When you go through your entire day hyperventilating and tensing your muscles, *without realizing it,* you've crossed the line from the "good" stress to the "bad" stress that will, sooner or later, break you down. The point of these exercises is to relearn what "normal" should feel like.

Relaxed, deep breathing is the key to breaking free of that stressed-out feeling when it hits. It may sound ridiculously easy, but in our text-message-a-minute world, you probably need to practice. The breathing exercise we offer becomes the foundation for the more advanced techniques that follow. With patients who like the feeling of "doing" something, we'll sometimes use the *body scan technique*. Taking "inventory" by concentrating on relaxing each part of your body in turn can be a great way to feel as if you are exercising control (or taking control back from chronic pain). With patients who are comfortable with the idea of completely "letting go," we might use a more "classical" meditation exercise where you focus on the breath and let your attention go wherever it wants before coming back to the breath (see the exercises in the box on pages 36–37).

These exercises may work directly on the source of the muscle pain, reducing it by reducing muscle tension. But they can also work indirectly, changing the way you experience pain. Okay, that may sound a little far-out. But pain isn't a solid, objective *thing*. It's the result of a conversation between special pain-sensing nerve cells spread throughout the body and a set of nerve cells housed in the spinal cord that send the information up to the brain to make sense of it all.

When you do a body scan or meditate, you're encouraging your body and mind to come to the calmest, coolest conclusion about the intensity of your muscle pain. The body is relaxed; the mind is focused on the present moment. Often, patients who deal with chronic muscle pain say their perception of it is driven as much by the fear that the pain will become intolerable as it is by the physical sensation itself. As someone once said, "Pain is inevitable; suffering is optional."

And as we'll detail in chapter 6, some of us would rather put the meditation cushion in the closet and go for a three-mile jog. Why not? It clears the mind and pumps up the good-feeling endorphins. No one mind-body approach is perfect for everybody. We have patients who have benefited from taking classes in Alexander Technique and Feldenkrais Method, two systems that bring awareness and disciplined training to a whole range of body movements.

Yoga is probably the most popular of these movement-based mind-body disciplines that we've encountered. In theory, we're all for it. Many of our patients use yoga as a rejuvenating break in their day or week. But some are borderline fanatic, pushing themselves into poses that are too aggressive or held too long. We see a lot of yoga-related injuries. If you're going to make use of Eastern mind-body techniques, check your "more is better" Western mind-set at the door. And know that although your limber friend on the next yoga mat may love certain poses, if you have spinal issues, they may not be right for you. You may benefit from the gentler movements of tai chi. Research any physical limitations you have and choose activities that best suit you.

SELF-DEFENSE

STRESS REDUCTION

Breathing Exercise (5–10 minutes daily)

Try this exercise for a week and see whether it makes a difference in your life. Find a quiet place and comfortable position, either sitting in a chair (spine straight, shoulders down and relaxed) or lying down. Close your eyes if that feels comfortable and doesn't send you to sleep. Bring all your attention to your breath. Concentrate on the in-breath, concentrate on the out-breath. The rhythm should be regular and relaxed. Don't exaggerate the slowness or the deepness of your breath. Relax your belly. You may be able to feel the belly rise and fall with each breath. (Don't worry if this "breathing from the diaphragm" doesn't come right away. Most people have unconsciously trained themselves to breathe more shallowly from the chest.) Each time your mind wanders, bring it back to the breath without judgment or frustration.

Body Scan Exercise (5–20 minutes daily, or as often as you find it useful)

Lie on your back on your bed or a foam pad on the floor. Close your eyes and concentrate on your breath, the rising and falling of your belly. After your breath has settled, feel your whole body, head to toe. Feel the parts of your body that are in contact with the bed or pad. Then bring your attention to the toes of your left foot. Feel every sensation going on there, good, bad, or indifferent. Then take a deeper breath, to "wash away" the toes, and move down to the heel of the foot. In this way, cover every region of your body. When your mind wanders, bring it back without judgment or frustration to the breath and to the part of the body that you are focusing your attention on. You may want to bring an element of visualization to this exercise. Picture the breath coming in through the nose, traveling to the body area, then running back out through the nose.

If you are in pain, you might imagine refreshing water or a healing light or a cool breeze traveling to the damaged area, bathing it, then leaving the body.

Meditation Exercise (5–30 minutes daily, or as consistently as you can manage)
If you find that meditation agrees with you, see if you can build up the duration of each session to twenty or thirty minutes, and if you can do it without strain and without its becoming the point of the exercise. To begin, assume a comfortable sitting or kneeling position on cushions or sit upright in a chair (spine straight, shoulders down). If you can maintain alertness, close your eyes. Bring your attention to your breath, the in-breath and the out-breath, the feeling of air passing through your nostrils, the rising and falling of your relaxed belly. When your mind wanders, note the thought or the feeling that comes into your head, then without judgment or frustration come back to the breath. If you are aware of physical discomfort or pain, bring your attention to that for a moment. Don't tell yourself a story about how you feel about the pain, just be fully in touch with the sensation, then return to the breath.

5

NUTRITION

Nutrition, the food choices you make every day, can affect the health and durability of your musculoskeletal system, and body weight can determine how durable that system needs to be. Quite possibly the single best thing you can do to preserve the long-term health of your joints is to keep your weight under control. You've got to manage the load you're asking your joints to carry. If you control the number of calories coming into the system so you *don't* put on that extra ten, or fifty, pounds when you hit your middle years, you can significantly lower your odds of developing osteoarthritis or suffering a traumatic cartilage injury (see the box on page 39). (Recall that when you climb stairs, every extra pound of weight exerts three to four extra pounds of pressure on your knees.)

The other part of the equation is how strong and resilient your body frame is in the first place. Here, you need to pay attention to the quality, not just the number, of the calories coming in. As we'll discuss, taking in the recommended amount of calcium and vitamin D preserves bone strength, and taking extra care to get "good" fat in your diet (the omega-3s) may protect against inflammation.

TALE OF THE TAPE MEASURE

Let's tackle weight first, specifically being overweight. Since the mid-1970s, the percentage of obese Americans has doubled. That's not good.

The physics of weight are pretty simple. Take in as many calories as you burn and you'll maintain your weight; take in fewer and you'll lose pounds. But if you struggle with weight, how do you consume fewer calories than your stomach wants without feeling cheated? Everyone who has ever seriously researched the subject (as opposed to churning out a diet bestseller) knows that crash diets don't work. In fact, most diets don't work. Motivated dieters can lose the weight, but their bodies, and psyches, can't handle the long-term deprivation, and they usually gain most or all of the pounds back. The key is sustainability. Forget about "going" on a diet as if it were a temporary fix. If you can consume fewer, but more nutritious, calories and burn more calories with a metabolism-revving exercise program such as the one we present in the next chapter, *and like this healthier lifestyle well enough to stick with it for the rest of your life,* then permanent weight loss *is* possible. As for an exact recipe for cutting calories without feeling intolerably hungry, if there were such a thing as a magic diet, science, or one very rich diet guru, would have found it by now. Follow your own stomach. Some people don't feel depleted when they take in fewer carbohydrates; others can go low-fat without feeling pleasure-starved.

INFO

WEIGHT AND JOINTS

According to a 2003 study in *Obesity Research* that looked at fifty-seven hundred Americans over the age of sixty, 56 percent of severely obese people had significant knee pain compared to 15 percent of the normal-weight group. In another recent study, severely obese women were twenty-five times more likely to suffer torn cartilage than their normal-weight counterparts; severely obese men were fifteen times as likely.

WHAT TO EAT: THE GOOD, THE BAD, AND THE UGLY

So, what to eat? Fortunately for us, there isn't one way to eat to control weight, another way to support bones and muscles, and another to fight disease. Healthy eating is healthy across the board. In the past decade, scientists have arrived at a consensus about what an optimal diet should look like. The two diets that have been most intensively studied, and heartily endorsed by researchers, the Mediterranean and the DASH (Dietary Approaches to Stop Hypertension), dovetail on the basics: heavy on whole grains, fruits, and vegetables, and light on sugar, salt, and animal fat. (The DASH emphasizes calcium, which, as we'll discuss, is good for the musculoskeletal system.)

Let's break it down. Everything you consume falls into three categories. Protein provides the building blocks for muscle growth and repair, and for the functioning of the immune system. Carbohydrates are fuel—your body breaks them down into simple sugars that are burned for energy. Fats provide essential lipids for the production of cell membranes and hormones, and allow the absorption of fat-soluble vitamins.

MINDFUL EATING

SELF-DEFENSE

Stop eating when you're no longer hungry. Considering seconds? Wait ten or twenty minutes until your stomach sensors have had time to register fullness.

Eat a nutritious appetizer such as soup or a salad before the entrée.

Use smaller plates. We're serious. Portion control works.

Spread out your calorie intake over the day with a high-quality midmorning and/or midafternoon snack such as yogurt, peanut butter, or a banana.

Proteins, carbs, and fat—all are essential parts of our diet, despite what you may have picked up from an endless stream of articles about low-fat versus low-carb strategies for losing weight. Healthy eating is all about appreciating that "good" proteins, carbs, and fats should be the cornerstones of your diet, and their "bad" evil twins should be eaten only in moderation or reserved for the occasional splurge.

Good protein delivers those necessary amino acids (from which the body builds new cells and repairs old ones) with a minimum of high-fat, high-calorie baggage.

Poultry (without the skin) is an excellent low-fat protein mainstay, as are low- or no-fat dairy products. But if you like red meat, there's no reason why you have to eliminate it altogether. A smallish five-ounce serving of a lean cut such as sirloin translates to fifteen grams of fat, which should fit almost anybody's daily nutritional budget. On the other hand, ten ounces of spareribs equals eighty grams of fat. You do the math.

Good carbohydrates are for the most part "complex" carbs, such as grains, fruits, and veggies, which are packed with fiber and water, which slow down digestion. Not only do these foods provide a nice, even energy flow over the day, they're packed with vitamins, minerals, and disease-fighting compounds. Sometimes the term *volumetrics* is used to describe the weight-control strategy of eating high-quality, high-bulk foods that fill you up without adding too many calories.

The "evil twin" carbs are the simpler ones that your body can most quickly break down and use as fuel. Sweets, snacks, and drinks laced with corn-syrup sweetener are one example. Starchy food with the fiber processed out of it—white bread, white rice, white pasta—is another. Simply put, whole foods are good, the refined, processed versions are not. When the simple carbs hit your system, blood sugar levels rise quickly and dramatically, stimulating your body to produce correspondingly high levels of insulin to clear the sugars out of the bloodstream and get them into muscle and liver cells for short-term storage. You may feel a boom-bust effect, a sugar rush followed by a feeling of fatigue or depletion. Over time, you can overstress your insulin system, leading to insulin resistance and, in serious cases, adult-onset diabetes.

As recently as fifteen years ago, all fat seemed to come in one flavor—bad. Weight-loss gurus and academic experts alike agreed that dietary fat—which packs nine calories per gram compared to four for carbohydrates and protein—was the major culprit behind heart disease and the ever-expanding American waistline. That was then. Now we appreciate the role of "good" fats in the diet. Monounsaturated fats, found in olive oil, canola oil, avocados, and nuts, helps lower LDL (low-density lipoprotein), the so-called bad cholesterol, and offers protection against disease. Polyunsaturated fats contain essential fatty acids that the body needs but does not itself produce. The omega-3 fatty acids are the stars of this group—they lower bad cholesterol and can reduce tissue inflammation, which explains why they seem to protect against diseases as various as heart disease, Alzheimer's, and arthritis. The most plentiful source of omega-3s is cold-water fish, but because of well-founded concern about mercury toxicity, you're better off sticking with the small fry down on the food chain such as herring and sardines. Other options are the new fortified foods such as omega-3-fortified eggs and orange juice, or supplemental oil and gelcaps.

The fats that deserve their nasty reputation are saturated and trans fats, both of which raise levels of LDL cholesterol. (Interestingly, it turns out that the dietary cholesterol found in egg yolks doesn't have a pronounced effect on cholesterol levels in the blood and doesn't deserve most of its old bad rep.) You don't need a nutrition degree to know that chicken skin, beef fat, and dairy products such as full-fat milk, yogurt, and cheese are heavy in saturated fats. But your body does need a modest amount of saturated fat, so unless you're on a strict low-fat diet for a heart condition, you can partake sensibly, from time to time. "Bad" saturated fat does taste good and does promote a feeling of satiety.

About trans fat, we have nothing positive to say. Trans or partially hydrogenated fat is created when vegetable oil is hydrogenated or processed to stay solid at room temperature. It's in margarine and vegetable shortening, commercially produced baked goods, and junk food. It raises bad LDL cholesterol and lowers good HDL (high-density lipoprotein) cholesterol. Fortunately, trans fats' deservedly bad press has prompted quite a few manufacturers to reduce or eliminate it from their products, so it's not as ubiquitous as it once was. Still, it pays to eat defensively—check the labels in the supermarket or the convenience store, and not only for trans fat. If the product in question has a laundry list of hard-to-pronounce preservatives and artificial flavorings, keep moving down the aisle. Better yet, move over to the fresh-produce aisle.

TOXIC FOOD?

Food safety is a legitimate concern. Buying organic is an effective, if somewhat more expensive, way to reduce your exposure to potentially harmful chemicals in the food supply. An influential group of environmental researchers in Washington, D.C., has developed a list of fruits and vegetables, "the dirty dozen," that have the heaviest pesticide load when conventionally grown. Spend 10–50 percent more for the organic versions and you'll be getting the most safety bang for your organic buck (see the box at right). You may also want to consider organic milk, beef, and poultry, also 10–50 percent more expensive than their conventional counterparts, which eliminate the hormones and antibiotics.

You may have noticed that we've talked mostly about food quality, not quantity, which is an individual matter. But nutritionists have found that when people make thoughtful food choices, their diets usually land within the government's dietary guidelines—approximately 45–60 percent carbs, 20–35 percent fats, and 10–35 percent protein—without their having to patrol the supermarket with a set of scales and a pocket calculator. But healthy differences in preferences may be influenced by your genetics. (The Alaskan Inuit evolved to thrive on a diet that heavily featured seal blubber. You, probably, have not.)

THE DIRTY DOZEN

(Compiled by the Environmental Working Group)

Rank	Fruit or Veggie	Score
1	Peaches (worst)	100 (highest pesticide load)
2	Apples	96
3	Sweet bell peppers	86
4	Celery	85
5	Nectarines	84
6	Strawberries	83
7	Cherries	75
8	Lettuce	69
9	Grapes, imported	68
10	Pears	65
11	Spinach	60
12	Potatoes	58

THE WHEN OF EATING

We said at the outset that maintaining a healthy weight is all about balancing the calories you consume with the calories you burn (and we'll get to the "burn" in the exercise chapter, which comes next). One more factor can be important: the when of eating.

Our colleague nutritionist Heidi Skolnik works with the New York Giants players and New York–area women at the Women's Sports Medicine Center at Manhattan's Hospital for Special Surgery. As Skolnik tells her clients, the body will likely signal that it wants food about every three hours. Even if you eat three squares

NUTRITIONIST
HEIDI SKOLNIK

Whether you're in the boardroom or the locker room, you want to be strategic about how you fuel your mind and your body. Maybe you're not being put through grueling workouts every day, but you have to stay alert in afternoon meetings and keep your weight under control. Healthy snacking, and staying away from junk food, is key. That doesn't just happen. If you stock your refrigerator with five yogurts or five packets of trail mix for the week's snacks, you're a lot less likely to wind up eating junk food.

daily, you'll probably still get hungry between meals. Most people adopt one of two unconscious strategies. They tide themselves over with junk food—sodas, chips, a scone, whatever is handy. Clearly, an extra load of sugar and trans or saturated fat is a bad idea. Or people ignore the hunger pangs (fairly easy if you're busy at work) and compensate by eating more at lunch or dinner or by having a late-night snack. The large infusion of calories late at night can overwhelm the body's capacity to break down and use them, causing many of the calories to be converted into body fat for storage. The solution is having a mid-morning or afternoon snack: a banana with some peanut butter; a container of yogurt; or an apple with some cheese (see the box above). If you still crave a late-night snack, you'll be able to make it a small and reasonable one.

DRINK UP

Let's talk about hydration. Remember that time-honored advice to drink eight glasses of water a day? It's the scientific equivalent of an urban myth—you won't ever find a study that came up with that figure. But the general idea is correct—proper hydration is absolutely essential for every body process you can think of, including muscle function and the lubrication of joints. But it doesn't have to be water; with the exception of alcohol, any kind of fluid will do. The popular line that coffee, tea, and caffeinated soft drinks don't count because caffeine is a diuretic—that is, it promotes urination—is overblown. They count. The real problem with many of these drinks is the calories. Every week, people routinely consume gallons of soft drinks, fruit drinks, coffee drinks, flavored teas, smoothies, and enhanced waters, all of which do little to cut appetite and a lot to worsen the problem of an overweight America. And diet beverages may be no better, introducing possibly harmful chemicals to the body.

The National Academy of Sciences has come up with some fluid-intake benchmarks: most men should try to drink about 101 ounces a day, most women, about 74 ounces (based on each gender's average weight). But in the real world, how much you drink should depend on your size, your activity level, how much you sweat, and the climate you live in. A more useful guide is to take in fluids at regular intervals, before and after exercise, and whenever you feel the slightest bit thirsty. (You might want to taper off your consumption in the evening so you don't have to keep waking up to go to the bathroom.) If your urine is light-colored and plentiful, mission accomplished. If it's darkish in color, drink up.

EATING FOR YOUR MUSCULOSKELETAL SYSTEM

Skolnik advises both the Giants and her female clients at the Hospital for Special Surgery on eating habits to preserve musculoskeletal health for the long haul. For women entering the menopausal years and beyond, getting enough calcium to protect bone density and reduce the risk of osteoporosis is a special concern. (The government recommends 1,000 milligrams for adults ages nineteen to fifty, 1,200 milligrams for adults fifty-one or older, and 1,200–1,500 milligrams for postmenopausal women.) A diet with plenty of (mostly low-fat) dairy products should do the trick (see the box on page 46). If not, a calcium citrate supplement can make up the difference. Besides calcium's bone-strengthening properties, evidence suggests that it helps to regulate blood pressure, and intriguing, preliminary evidence suggests that it may stimulate the body to burn fat more efficiently. No matter how good you think your diet may be, if you're a woman over forty, you should get a bone-density test and a full blood and urine test workup to see if you're at risk for osteoporosis. Senior men can also be at risk.

It isn't enough just to consume calcium. The body has to properly absorb it, and here vitamin D plays a crucial role. During the warm-weather months, your body manufactures vitamin D when your skin is exposed to sunlight. During the colder months (or all year if you don't go outside much or wear strong sunblock re-

PUTTING CALCIUM IN YOUR DIET

(Chart figures mostly from USDA National Nutrient
Database for Standard References, Release 21)

Food	Amount	Calcium (mg)
Calcium-fortified cereal (brand: Total)	¾ cup	1,000
Yogurt, low-fat, plain	8 oz	415
Calcium-fortified orange juice	1 cup	350
Sardines	3 oz	325
Spinach, cooked	1 cup	291
Milk, low-fat	1 cup	290
Soy milk, fortified	1 cup	300
Cottage cheese, low-fat	1 cup	206
Chedder cheese, reduced-fat	1 oz	200
Salmon, canned, with bones	3 oz	181
Tofu, processed with calcium	¼ block	163
Almonds	⅓ cup	110
Beans, cooked	½ cup	25–65
Broccoli, cooked	1 cup	61

ligiously when you do), your stores of vitamin D drop. Foods such as organ meats and cold-water fish such as sardines and herring have some vitamin D, but you'd have to eat like a Siberian fisherman to reach the government's recommended daily intake of 400 international units. The usual route is fortified foods (milk is usually fortified with 125 IU) and supplements (a good multivitamin should have 400 IU, but make sure it's the more potent vitamin D3 form). Because a hip fracture can be a life-threatening trauma for the elderly, especially elderly women, Skolnik recommends for them a daily intake of at least 800 IU and, depending on the individual, as high as 2,000 IU. Have your vitamin D levels checked and consult with your doctor. (Vitamin D deficiency can result in muscle pain, and recent studies have linked low vitamin D intake with an increased risk of cancer, among other diseases. That should get your attention considering 41 percent of men and 53 percent of women in the United States are vitamin D deficient.)

Supplementing with omega-3 fatty acids to reduce inflammation and protect muscles and connective tissues is also a sensible choice. (Skolnik suggests a two-to-four-gram daily intake, taking the pill with food and splitting up the dosage over the day.)

There are other joint-friendly supplements out there with some supporting science on their side (if not the research pedigree of omega-3) that may be worth looking into. SAM-e (S-Adenosyl-methionine) is derived from the amino acid methionine; Zyflamend combines two spices with confirmed anti-inflammatory effects, ginger and turmeric. Enthusiasm, and positive study results, has waned for another combo supplement, glucosamine and chondroitin. In a 2006 *New England Journal of Medicine* study, the supplement did not reduce pain overall, but did benefit one subgroup of patients with moderate to severe pain. In a smaller 2008 study published in *Arthritis and Rheumatism*, the supplement scored no better than a sugar pill placebo. (Check with your physician before beginning any supplementation program.)

6

FITNESS

In the previous two chapters, we've discussed how to relax the body and how to fuel it. Now we're ready to take it out for a spin. If you're not exercising, we'll provide some safe, smart ways to get moving. If you're already a recreational athlete (a regular jogger or tennis player, for instance), we'll discuss how to modify your routine so you can perform at a satisfying level and minimize the chance of injury.

WHY EXERCISE?

Beginner or veteran athlete, you reap a host of physical benefits when you exercise. When you push your body against the "resistance" of gravity and the ground (walking, jogging, playing tennis, etc.) or your own weight (push-ups, pull-ups, etc.) or a piece of exercise equipment (rubber cables, elastic bands, dumbbells, free weights, weight machines), you stress your entire musculoskeletal system. Provided you don't overdo it and overwhelm the system, this is healthy stress. The blood pumps more vigorously, oxygenating your tissues; the synovial fluid that lubricates the joints gets a boost. Muscles, bones, and connective tissues adapt and become stronger and better able to handle the challenges of everyday life. Later in life, there's less chance of osteoporosis and bone breaks, less chance of taking a fall because your muscle strength or your balance fails you, and a greater chance of being able to right yourself if you do fall.

Body weight is an issue. Many people, especially in their middle years, have trouble maintaining a healthy weight through diet alone. Aerobic or endurance work is an excellent way to burn calories. And the muscle tissue you build doing strength work burns more calories than fat does, even at rest. (Only 4 more calories per pound per day, but it also increases the body's fat-burning potential.)

Exercisers carry many benefits with them into their middle and senior years. They are better able to avoid the extra pounds that are a risk factor for diabetes and heart disease. The aerobic exercise they do tones and strengthens the entire system: the heart beats more efficiently and the levels of HDL, the "good" cholesterol, go up, both of which protect against heart attack; and the cells stay more receptive to insulin, so the body is more resistant to diabetes. Some evidence even suggests that exercise can help ward off certain types of cancers.

THE EXCUSES

So why do half the people in America fail to meet the government recommendation of thirty minutes of moderate activity most days of the week. Let's put it another way: if you're in this camp, what's wrong with you? We don't have to read the latest government study to answer that one; we talk to our patients every day. In our experience, they fall into two groups. The first is the "it's hopeless" group: "Doctor, it's hopeless; my knee hurts so I can't run"; "My shoulder hurts so I can't swim"; "I've got an artificial knee so I can't exercise, and now I've gained weight so there's another reason I can't exercise." Our answer is, all people can do something if they're willing to push a bit beyond their comfort zone.

The key is starting small and building up as you can handle it. Consistency, getting into a groove and staying there, is more important than any single heroic performance that you'll have a tough time repeating. If you can't jog, swim. If you can't swim, ride a bicycle or a stationary exercise bike. If you can't do that, try one of those gym hand-bikes (arm ergometers), where you get the aerobic benefit by working your upper body, rotating the pedals with your hands. (American distance-running great Joan Benoit Samuelson had knee surgery two weeks before the 1984 Olympic marathon trials but was able to maintain her aerobic fitness on the hand-bike. She went on to win the women's marathon at both the trials and the Olympics.)

Our other nonexercisers tend to fall into the school of "the road to hell is paved with good intentions." They're the optimists who have every intention of rescheduling their lives around the exercise they never had time for before. "I'm going to join a gym near the office and work out every lunch hour" is a typical bold plan. Unfortunately, most people don't make the jump from sedentary to gym rat in one giant step, and most people's jobs are good at generating reasons for staying glued to the office chair. So start slow and, whenever possible, modify your routine, don't try to change it overnight. For example, you might set aside a half hour as soon as you get home from work to go on a brisk walk. It's likely you'll feel like going to bed earlier, you'll sleep more soundly, and life will seem better in the morning. This is a modified routine you can build on. (Check out the box on page 51 for more routine "tweaks.")

FREQUENCY, DURATION, INTENSITY

Let's assume you've taken the first step, invariably the hardest one, and have begun to get your body moving in your everyday life. Maybe you've always been an active person, but you've put on some pounds in your middle years and realize that it's time to invest more energy into your health and appearance. Either way, you're ready to integrate exercise into your life in a more systematic way.

So we'll provide you with a basic structure and some of our favorite exercises to help you get started. Pick and choose, and most definitely skip anything that is too demanding or stresses a vulnerable joint. (If you're not sure where to start, talk

BUILDING EXERCISE INTO YOUR DAY

Take the stairs instead of the elevator. After you've mastered the basics, you can take two stairs at a time to work on the quads, hams, and glutes (thighs and butt).

Park your car at the farthest-away spot in the lot. If you use public transportation, get on or off one stop beyond your usual stop.

At the office, walk down the hall and talk to someone instead of always sending e-mails.

Do your own housework; wash and dry dishes by hand.

Go back to the pushmower. For large lawn owners, reserve one section for the push-mower. Or grow a garden.

Go dancing. If you have thick curtains, dance at home.

it over with a physical therapist or a physician.) In the hot-spot chapters that follow, we'll tackle those physical vulnerabilities head-on. What we present here is a general framework for developing and maintaining lifelong fitness.

In the beginning, slow and steady wins every time. Consistency will get you greater fitness gains, with less chance of injury, than will a burst of activity one week and then none the next. You can't make up for lost time by simply doing more—the body can only adapt to so much before it breaks down. Remember, strength and flexibility must be balanced. For example, if you're flexible but your muscles aren't strong, that increased range of motion won't have much practical benefit and could lead to injury. By the same token, strength without flexibility is also of limited use. Some weight lifters can barely lift their arms over their head because they have failed to distribute that strength over a "functional" range of motion. All that strength, and they still can't put a box of light cereal away on the top shelf.

Any exercise program boils down to what you do and how you do it. The what of our plan is a combination of warm-up/balance, strength, cardio. The how is measured by three variables: frequency, or how often you work out; duration, or how long you work out; and intensity, or how hard you work out. At the beginning, be as consistent as you can be, four to six workouts a week if that's possible. But as you get familiar with this new routine, we want you to become mindful of those three hows—frequency, duration, intensity—so you can adapt your workouts to the requirements of your body and the demands of your life. Maybe you're feeling washed out at work. Then it's time to reduce one or two of those variables. On the other hand, maybe your energy is good but you've got a tough week coming up at the office that will limit the time you can spend working out. That's your cue to raise the intensity. If you can only spend twenty minutes in the gym or on the track, make them count, within the limits of safety and good sense.

With time and experience, you'll mix up the variables of your workouts not just because you need to but because you want to challenge your body in different ways. An unvarying routine is the enemy of improvement and a sure way to get bored or even injured. For instance, if you're a runner, instead of running the same medium-tempo five miles every day, you might want to devote one day a week to a longer run (duration), or one day to some sprints (intensity). If you do squats as a part of your strength-training regimen, one day you can do fewer repetitions with a heavier weight, and on another you can do a greater number of body-weight squats. Whether you're working on cardio, strength, or flexibility, don't overload your body in too many ways at once.

INFO

EXERCISE ON A TIME BUDGET

Even if you have limited time, you can still manage a concise, varied, successful exercise program, with both cardio and strength components. For instance, five minutes of warm-up/dynamic stretch, twenty minutes of cardio, twenty minutes of strength, and ten minutes of cooldown and dynamic or movement stretching. With just three to four days a week, for forty-five minutes to an hour, you can make some real progress. However, when you combine cardio and strength, you should do both with moderate intensity (55–70 percent of your maximum effort, for example). In an ideal world it is better to separate cardio and strength. Especially if you have specific performance goals, it may be harder to reach them with the intensity/duration limitations of a combined program. But you can definitely achieve overall fitness and balance.

THE ALL-PURPOSE FITNESS PLAN

Getting Started: Warm-up/stretching/balance/skill drills, five to twenty minutes, every day or as often as you can manage, and always before strength or cardio workouts.

Warm-up

Remember the time-honored advice to stretch before working out. Well, scratch that. What's more important is a five- to ten-minute warm-up to get the blood pumping to the muscles and to warm up the entire musculoskeletal system. As your body begins to generate heat, your connective tissue softens and becomes more pliable and less prone to strain, sprain, or tear. Outdoors, a brisk walk or a slow jog is a good option. At the gym, keeping a low intensity on the treadmill, elliptical trainer, or stationary bike all work just fine.

Stretching

As we'll discuss in the next chapter, a lot of exercise experts have grown skeptical about the benefits of "static" stretching, where you hold a stretch for ten to thirty seconds. But "dynamic" stretching, where you incorporate movement, is a good way to stimulate the muscle to recover its full, natural range of motion. There is no one perfect time to stretch. Anytime after the warm-up is fine. Some runners may discover that they get more benefit from stretching after their run to relieve tightness in their calf muscles. Try some of these dynamic movements to see what works for you:

- Extend your arms sideways and move them around in a circle. Start with small, tight circles and expand. Switch to your legs. Balance on one leg, lift the other slightly in front of you, and rotate it as though you were trying to draw a circle with your foot. Change legs.
- Vigorously move your outstretched arms from the front to the side and back, crisscrossing the arms in front of the chest.
- Hold on to a table or a fence or a pole with your left arm and swing your right leg and right arm in the opposite direction, loose and easy. Change sides.
- Lie on the floor on your back, knees bent, feet flat on the ground. Keeping the knees together, lower them both to one side. Then, engaging the abs, swing the knees to the other side. Go back and forth in a continuous movement.

Balance

In bare feet, stand on one leg for twenty seconds, then switch to the other leg for twenty seconds. (If you start to lose your balance, stop and start over again; don't wave your arms around to try to recover.) To make it more challenging, switch back to the original leg and balance for twenty seconds, this time with your eyes closed, then back to the other leg for twenty seconds, eyes closed. Not only are you working the postural muscles to keep you upright without the usual support (i.e., two legs), the eyes-closed portion trains mind and body to know where you are in space (i.e., proprioception), and to stay in balance without visual cues.

The single-leg toe touch is a great all-in-one exercise that strengthens the muscles of the entire body, including the core, as they help with balance and stabilization. If you're not ready for it now, come back to it in a few weeks or months. Stand balanced on one foot, keeping the back and neck in a straight line. Keep your eyes fixed on a point on the floor about four feet in front of your foot. Bend at the waist, reaching for the supporting foot with the opposite hand. Bend the knee as much as necessary to balance and stay pain-free. Hold for a count of two. Do ten repetitions, held for no more than two seconds each. The goal is not to reach the foot but to stay steady. Remember to breathe and not clench the teeth. (See page 167.)

The yoga "sun salutation" is another excellent combination of balance, stretch, and strength. With twelve distinct movements in a sequence, the how-to is a little cumbersome, but you can Google the instructions or buy a beginner's yoga book or, better yet, take a class. (You could think of it as a more "mindful" Eastern version of stretch, push-up, and squat-thrust rolled into one.) Five or ten sun salutations will prime the body for just about any workout.

Skill

The problem with out-of-condition recreational athletes is that too often they think they're still young, conditioned athletes. That's how they persuade themselves that it's okay to jump back into a softball or basketball league, or a regular tennis routine, and not suffer any ill effects even though they've been out of the game for years or decades. If you're serious about not hurting yourself, you should spend two to four weeks on conditioning and technique before you ever set foot on the court or in the batter's box. Every workout should include ten to twenty minutes spent on technique and coordination. For instance, softball players need to spend time in the batting cage and running the base paths. Basketball players might do a "hopping" drill like this: balance on the left leg and hop forward, landing on the right leg and balance for two seconds; hop back onto the left leg and repeat five to ten times. Runners should do lateral movement exercises (for instance, skip sideways without crossing your legs) to build up the muscles that running doesn't develop. Tennis players and golfers should build in time for regular "touch-up" sessions with a teaching pro. Rarely do topflight tennis players and golfers suffer from tennis elbow and golfer's elbow (see chapter 10 for that discussion). These overuse injuries are usually the result of an amateur's bad form, which can and should be corrected.

Strength: Fifteen to forty minutes, two to four times a week.

Building a Strength Program

Here, we provide a menu of exercises; you build a program that works for you. But some general rules do apply. Unless you're working toward a specific goal with a personal trainer, there's no need to do strength workouts more often than every other day. You're stressing muscles that need time to rebuild and rebound. In general, we'd like you to do at least one exercise from each of the three groups— upper body, core, lower body—and an all-body exercise if you're so inspired. Don't push yourself to the point where your good form breaks down. That's inviting injury, not protecting against it. A useful rule of thumb is, stop when you feel you've got two more repetitions left in you (e.g., if you could squeeze out seven push-ups, do five for one set). As for the number of sets per exercise, two or three sets would be ideal, but one set is a lot better than none. People's goals will differ. Some people will want to reach a "base level" of fitness and maintain it from there. Others will want to continue to get stronger, which means, at some point, they'll need a wider selection of exercises to stress the body in different ways. Find a good trainer!

Upper Body

In life, the one weight that we must be able to handle is our own body. That's why we love the classic body-weight exercises for all-around fitness such as the push-up and the pull-up. Forget how many you can do, perfect form is everything. Even if you have been doing these exercises for years, you can always reassess and tweak your form.

The ideal push-up: Assume the familiar prone push-up position. Your feet should be about shoulder-width apart with your hands braced on the floor, next to your shoulders. The shoulders and upper back should be pulled back and "down," not hunched up or rounded. First make sure you can hold that raised push-up position: arms straight, face down with neck in a straight, "neutral" position, back flat, abs held in, no sagging the hips. You may feel your ab muscles shaking after a few seconds! Then slowly lower your body (count to three) as one unit, leading with your chest, until your elbows are at ninety degrees and hold for a count of one. Come back up to the starting position, counting one or two. Inhale on the way down, exhale on the way up. Your abdominal muscles should be firing the whole time, helping to keep your body straight. Repeat as many times as you can comfortably manage with good form. Bad form is letting your midsection drop, not going low enough, or moving your hands forward and hunching your shoulders. The motion should be slow and controlled, not fast and sloppy.

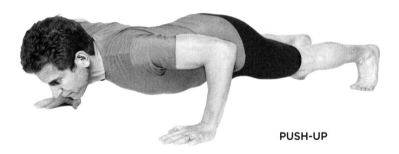

PUSH-UP

Lots of people can't do one proper push-up. Doing push-ups from the knees-down position is a common modification, but we prefer staying in the straight-line position and doing the push-ups against an angled surface, for instance, hands braced on the kitchen counter, the stairs, or a park bench. Seniors with physical limitations can do them from a standing position, against the wall. With your arms fully extended and hands flat against the wall or bench in front of you, relax your elbows and lean into the wall or bench. Then push back to your starting position, keeping your body straight the whole time. This doubles as a good exercise to develop the strength and the reflexes needed to break a fall with the hands and arms.

Push-ups can be made tougher as well. Modify the starting position by bringing the feet closer together or drop your chest closer to the floor. Do the push-up with one foot off the ground or with both feet raised, resting on a chair, bench, or a stability ball.

The ideal pull-up: Not too many people have a pull-up bar bolted to a wall at home, so you'll likely have to visit a local playground or make the trip to the gym. Grip the bar with the palms facing out and the hands a little wider than shoulders' width apart. The arms should be straight at the start of the movement, whether you are hanging or using a support. Tighten your ab muscles, keep the shoulder blades together and down, and then slowly pull your body up as you count to one or two, leading with the chest and squeezing the shoulders back. Exhale at the top. Your chin should clear the bar, but do not jut it forward or pull yourself forward over the bar. Hold for one count, then, inhaling, lower yourself to a three count. Keep your

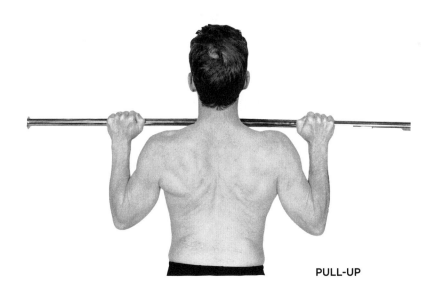

PULL-UP

shoulders back and down and do not round your back or shoulders! You may find it easier to stay in balance by crossing your ankles and flexing your knees. Stop before your form begins to crumble.

Lots of people can't do a single proper pull-up. No shame there. Find a low, chest-height playground bar. Standing with your chest next to the bar, grasp the bar and lean backward until your arms are fully extended. To make it harder, move your feet farther in front of the bar so your body is at a steeper angle. Pull yourself toward the bar until your chest touches it, and repeat for the number of repetitions in your set. An even better solution is the Gravitron machine at the gym, which uses a counterweight system to let you adjust the amount of resistance as you move your body up and down. There are several grips so you can work a range of muscles.

Core

The plank: This is one of the best, and simplest, ways to work the abdominal muscles. Assume the prone push-up position, but with your weight on your forearms, elbows bent at about forty-five degrees, and hands angling in toward the center, in a fist position, thumbs-up. Keep the shoulders down, back straight, hips up, and hold the position as long as you can maintain good form. Try fifteen, then thirty, then forty-five seconds, and so on. You can further increase the burn by resting your forearms on a stability ball. To work the oblique abdominal muscles, switch to a side-plank position. Lie on your side and elevate youself by putting your weight on one forearm, perpendicular to the body, elbow bent at ninety degrees. Your legs are stacked one on top of the other; the hand of your non-weight-bearing arm is resting on your raised hip. Hold the pose as long as you can keep your body in a still, straight line. Switch sides and repeat. (See pages 163 snd 164.)

Stability-ball crunch: Probably the most common core exercise. The standard crunch is not your only option. It doesn't target the core as a unit, you can cheat with body momentum, and it can stress the neck. A better option is the stability-ball crunch. Stretch your back out on a stability ball. With your knees bent and feet planted on the floor, lift your shoulder blades off the ball, two or three counts coming up, the same coming down. Five or ten stability-ball crunches can work your abs more thoroughly than as many or more "classic" crunches. (See page 165.)

The stability ball, however, can be very challenging for those with back and neck issues or balancing issues. An alternative is a variation on the standard floor crunch. Lying on your back, bend your knees slightly to take the pressure off your lower back. Put your hands by your ears (without pushing your head forward) and lift your upper body slightly off the ground by contracting your abs and bringing your chest toward the ceiling. If your neck feels strained, use your hands and fingertips to support your head, taking pressure off your neck.

Dead bug: Here's an alternative to the stability-ball crunch that's better for people with neck- or shoulder-muscle issues, the easy-to-remember Dead bug. Lie on your back, keeping the spine neutral at all times. Bring both feet up, knees directly over your hips and bent at a ninety-degree angle. Raise both arms, then extend your left arm straight back behind you and at the same time drop your right heel and extend your right leg straight out, hovering just above the ground. Keep your abdominal muscles engaged. Then slowly bring your legs and arms back to the starting position and repeat, this time extending the right arm behind and the left leg in front. Do as many repetitions as you can manage with good form, keeping your abs engaged and back flat against the floor. Only lower your arms and legs as far as you can with control.

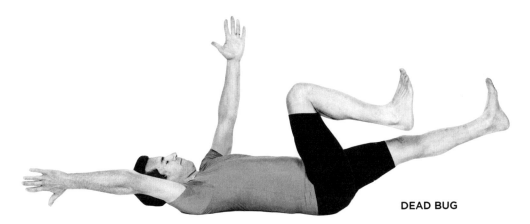

DEAD BUG

Superman: This is a great exercise to work the abdominals and the lower-back muscles. Lie facedown on a mat or some other forgiving flat surface with your legs together. Extend your arms behind you, keeping them close by your sides, with your palms facing up and thumbs pointing up. Extend and lift your torso at the waist, so your arms, chest, and torso all lift off the ground. Keep your neck straight, your head in a "neutral" position, and your shoulder blades squeezed together and away from your ears. Hold the pose for thirty to forty-five seconds or as long as you can manage with good form, then relax and repeat. (See page 162.)

Lower Body

Body-weight squats: This is a great workout for the core and lower body. Stand with your feet slightly wider than shoulders' width apart. Hold your hands out in front of you, on your hips, or behind your head. Keeping a straight back, bend the knees, lowering the buttocks toward the floor until the hip reaches knee level, or as far as it is possible to go with good form and no pain. Sit back so that your knees do not go past your toes. Contract the ab and butt muscles and bring yourself to a standing position. Do ten repetitions, holding for no more than two seconds each. (See page 194.)

Step-ups: Stand in front of a box or a bench, anywhere from half a foot to a foot and a half high, depending on your level of fitness. With your hands on your hips and your back straight, step up with your left foot, then bring your right foot up, then step down in the same order. Repeat, leading with the right foot, then alternate. You can make the exercise more challenging by holding your hands behind your head.

Body-weight lunges: Stand straight with your feet slightly less than shoulders' width apart, hands on your hips. Take a big step forward, with the knee of your leading leg bent ninety degrees, your back leg slightly flexed, heel off the ground, weight on the ball of the foot. Return to the starting position and step forward with the other leg then alternate. Create a right angle with the front hip and knee—in other words, don't let the knee go past the toe.

All Body

Wood chop: Here's a simple routine that works several muscle groups at once. With your legs shoulders' width apart, hold a weighted ball at chest level. Lift the ball over your head, then, while bending your knees, bring it down between your knees, then back overhead as you straighten your legs. Do five to ten repetitions. For extra credit, include spinal rotators: do the same number of reps, only this time bring the ball down to your right knee and then back over to your left ear, then down to your left knee and up over to the right ear.

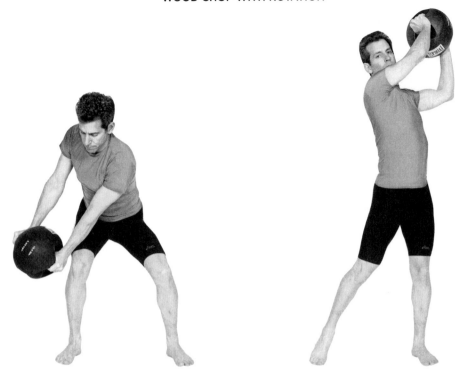

Ball toss-up: Keeping your elbows in, toss a basketball (or any ball with some heft) up against a wall about a foot or two above your head. Catch it and repeat fifteen to thirty times or as many times as you can comfortably manage. To work more muscle groups and add difficulty to an already deceptively demanding exercise, catch the ball, squat, return to standing, then toss it up again. (We discovered this one at www.crossfit.com, a great source of fun and effective exercise ideas.)

Cardio: Twenty to sixty minutes, three to six times a week.

Duty and obligation may bring you to the treadmill or the elliptical trainer, but they won't necessarily keep you there. That's why we're big believers in building a cardio/aerobic program around something you love to do. It doesn't matter whether your chosen activity is purely aerobic such as jogging and cycling, or a "skill" sport that requires a lot of running around such as basketball and the racquet sports. It all counts. (Sorry, golfers and softball players are going to have supplement with something more vigorous.) Look around and you'll notice that the people who maintain their fitness year in and year out are the ones who have their "thing."

But don't make the mistake of thinking you can play your way back into shape. If you don't have a decent aerobic conditioning base, you're putting yourself at risk by running around the basketball or tennis court once or twice a week. It's back to Cardio 101 for you.

Cardio 101
(Red flag: Get clearance from your doctor
before beginning a cardio program)

If you're new to cardio work or have been away so long you might as well be new, pick a sport or an activity that you think might appeal to you. If you have no physical limitations, the field is wide-open. If, however, knee trouble runs in your family and you've got the beginnings of osteoarthritis, regular jogging isn't a good bet, nor, for that matter, is any jarring activity that sends impact shock to the knee. Walking, the elliptical trainer, swimming, aqua aerobics/"water jogging," and cycling are all sensible choices.

Next, you need to develop a base of endurance fitness, slowly and surely so as not to overtax the muscles, connective tissues, or the heart. Here, we recommend a "walk/run" approach, a concept we learned from the well-known running educator Jeff Galloway and modified for beginners and recreational runners coming off injuries. The concept is simple and can be applied to any form of endurance exercise: basically, alternate periods of low- and medium-intensity effort. Your doctor should advise you on the intensity levels for your beginner's program, but here's a typical program. Start with approximately ten minutes of low-intensity warm-up at 50–60 percent of maximum heart rate (if you've got a heart-rate monitor) or 5–6 on a 10-point "perceived effort" scale (if you don't). That's followed by one minute of moderate-intensity work (60–70 percent of maximum heart rate or 6–7 perceived effort), then one minute of low-intensity work. These rounds of low- and medium-intensity exercise alternate for as many as ten cycles, depending on the length you choose for your workout. End with a ten-minute, cooldown low-intensity walk (or cycle or swim).

If you can comfortably handle this routine after a week or two, then bump it up: the opening ten-minute walk followed by alternating rounds of two-minute moderate-intensity runs and one-minute walks, then the ten-minute cooldown. As your cardiovascular system gets stronger and more efficient (and injuries, if you have them, heal), you can work through the program all the way to alternating rounds of fifteen-minute runs and one-minute walks. After developing a good aerobic base, recreational athletes whose sports require short bursts of intense effort should also devote one or two workouts a week that include ten to forty minutes in the higher-effort zone (an example might be 70–90 percent of maximum heart rate or 7–9 perceived effort) to train their cardiovascular system to handle those stiffer demands. Sprints, short ten-second-to-one-minute bursts on the cardio machine, sprinting against high resistance in a cycling class, or hill-climbing on a real bike— they all work.

Of all the aerobic sports we've discussed, running—the impact of all those foot

SELF-DEFENSE

RUNNING

Running can be a wonderful way to exercise while enjoying the outdoors or the company of friends, but it can also create or aggravate injuries and weaknesses. Over time the accumulated impact shock of intensive long-distance running will likely take a toll on your entire lower body, not just your knees. (If you don't believe us, ask some of the distance running stars of the seventies and eighties who built their careers on hundred-mile-a-week-plus training.) You can earn almost all of running's cardiovascular health gains with only moderate distance work, twenty to thirty miles a week. So be smart. Don't overdo the hill workouts that place extra stress on the knees, especially the running-downhill part. Try to run on softer surfaces and avoid running on crowned roads where your "downhill" leg is stressed by the slope. Consider a run/walk program or strategy. If you're over thirty or thirty-five and you're not training for competition, there's no need to run more than every other day—your muscles and connective tissues need time to recover. Cross-training with sports such as cycling and swimming that are easier on the joints and muscles is an excellent way to maintain aerobic fitness on the off days and to avoid burnout. Make sure your running shoes fit properly and replace them every five hundred miles or so, or every six months, whichever milestone you hit first. (From constant pounding, or just from the passage of time, the air-cell foam in the inner soles hardens.)

strikes—places tremendous demands on the legs and the core muscles (see the box on page 63). Even if you are in great cardiovascular shape, it's still a smart injury-prevention strategy to slow down at regular intervals and walk for thirty seconds or a minute. Listen to your body, and walk after every lap, mile, or five minutes of running time—whatever feels right for you. By giving the muscles a chance to

SURVIVING THE GYM

You'll notice that none of the exercises we offer require you go to a health-club gym. A well-equipped gym is a good place to work out, but don't pin all your hopes on it if you don't have the schedule or the self-discipline to make it there three to five times a week. We actually prefer the body-weight-resistance exercises you can do at home to the weight machines at the gym. Exercises such as the basic push-up or the pull-up don't isolate one set of muscles like many gym machines. They work a bunch of different muscle groups (the push-up develops the pectorals, biceps, triceps, shoulder muscles, abdominals, back-stabilizing muscles, etc.), all of which lead to better, more functional, all-round fitness. As you recall from chapter 2, muscles work in tandem, agonist and antagonist. If you're pumping up your quadriceps on the leg-extension machine and ignoring the hamstrings, you're creating muscle imbalances that can increase the odds of injury.

In your average gym, people often "cheat" by using momentum to lift weights that are too heavy for them. This herky-jerky approach risks injury and defeats the point of the exercise, which should be to develop muscle strength evenly across the joint's range of motion. The best way to achieve this is by focusing on a slow, controlled motion as you lift the weight up (concentric motion) and lower it down (eccentric motion), whether you're pushing a barbell or your own body weight.

If you are going the gym route and you're not well versed in the proper techniques for the latest gym equipment, get a trainer, at least to get started. And not just any trainer, but one who is sympathetic to your goals. If you're a fifty-year-old woman who wants help losing ten pounds and building up some lean-muscle mass, and the first trainer you come across only wants to do Olympic weight lifting, keep looking. Assuming that any health-club trainer should be able to customize a program to meet your needs may be setting yourself up for disappointment.

relax, you can cut down on the incidence of strains to the Achilles tendon, calf, hamstring, and abdominal muscles that are the bane of the sport. At twenty, this kind of "defensive" running probably isn't necessary for most people. At forty, it could be what keeps you in the jogging game.

Advanced Cardio

Getting in shape is one thing, keeping fit is another. For the serious recreational endurance athlete who's been running or cycling or swimming for years, we offer some hard-won advice about keeping it going in a fun and healthy way that we've drawn from our own experience and from friends and patients such as Mike Llerandi, who for the past twenty years has been one of the country's top amateur triathletes.

Mike's philosophy of training and aging is "adapt, don't concede." As your family and work responsibilities likely increase in your thirties, forties, and beyond, make good use of your weekends. If, for example, you can fit in a two or three-hour bike ride on a Saturday or Sunday, you can use the workweek for shorter, brisker rides and still be able to cycle at a fairly high level. As much as possible, integrate your family and social life with your athletic one. The Llerandi gold standard? Try to do at least one weekly workout with your spouse. You may have to back off on the intensity or duration (possibly not a bad thing), but you may get a less stressful life and a better marriage. Kids can be brought into the act as well. (For several years, Mike's daughter accompanied him on his training runs on her bike, handing him the water bottle when he needed it.) Having one or more friends with whom you regularly run or cycle or swim is a huge plus. Not only does a group ensure that the workouts actually take place, but they'll also be more fun, with a jolt of competitive energy.

You need to assess your own (aging) body with the same practical realism that you bring to balancing life and training. Workouts that might have seemed routine in your twenties are likely to break you down in your forties. Overtraining can show up in subtle ways (trouble sleeping, bad mood, greater-than-expected muscle soreness) and not so subtle ways (injury), so it pays to be vigilant. Again, adapt, don't concede. Take a hard look at those three variables of your training schedule—

intensity, duration, and frequency—and see what you need to modify to stay fresh. Because the body of the older athlete requires more time to recover after a hard effort, the three variables of training may need to be downscaled.

Few runners or cyclists or swimmers in their forties and older can pack in more than one weekly workout at all-out levels of exertion without eventually running out of gas or getting injured. Whether you're a masters-level competitor or just someone who values his or her fitness, most of your training should be spent in a comfortable aerobic zone: 65–75 percent of maximum heart rate or approximately 6.5–7.5 perceived effort.

Cross-training is the safe way to keep your workout frequency high, up to five or six sessions a week. With different sports, you're working different and often complementary muscle groups so you're less prone to muscle overload or imbalance injuries. Running and cycling, running and swimming, and cycling and swimming are all great pairs. Of course, in theory you could still overdo the cardio intensity with a mix of sports, but in practice runners tend to go at a saner pace on the bike as do cyclists when they run.

Maybe the hardest thing the recreational athlete must do is to junk the philosophy of "no pain, no gain." A good workout isn't the one that leaves you feeling wiped out. Finishing a workout feeling relaxed and refreshed is the winning strategy in the long run. Consider yourself in training for the big event, otherwise known as life.

In chapters 8–14, we divide up the body into seven "hot spots"—neck, shoulder, elbow/wrist/hand, lower back, hip, knee, ankle and foot—where most musculoskeletal trouble turns up. All the damage we discuss is divided into three categories: Mostly Muscular; Muscle or Joint?; Joint/Orthopedic. The first and maybe most important thing we do is figure out how the three elements of the system—muscle, joint, bone—may be out of sync. (In some cases, nerve injury becomes a contributing factor.) Always, we treat as conservatively as possible, working first on the muscles if there's a reasonable chance to fix the problem without drugs or surgery. Keep in mind, this book is a practical guide that covers many of the most common musculoskeletal problems, not a comprehensive orthopedic or therapeutic manual. If you have a serious injury, get help from a health professional.

At the end of each of these chapters, we hand you the tools of muscle medicine, taking you through our self-treatment program of hands-on self-treatment techniques, stretching, and strengthening, introduced here in chapter 7.

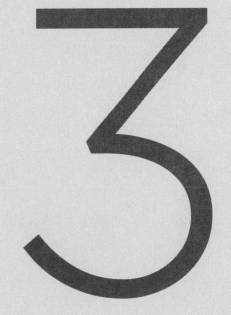

PART

3

TROUBLESHOOTING YOUR MUSCLES: THE "HOT SPOTS"

THE MUSCLE MEDICINE PROGRAM

In our era, there's no shortage of musculoskeletal expertise, from high-tech surgical advances to the latest variation of hands-on therapeutic techniques. The problem is, unlike in other areas of health care, a consistent strategy that governs how and when people receive treatment for their musculoskeletal problems is often lacking.

We'll frequently see people with tight or inflamed muscles doing muscle conditioning work in physical therapy, but not getting better and putting themselves at risk for reinjury. Right therapy, wrong timing. The piece of the puzzle that's sometimes missing is the treatment of those tight and injured muscles beforehand. You can't stretch and strengthen damaged tissue (only the healthy tissue around it), but you can further irritate it.

THE STRATEGY

Over the past six years, combining forces to deal with our patients' musculoskeletal problems and following their progress, or sometimes lack of progress, in therapy, we've developed our own treatment strategy. Whether the patient is in prehab to prepare for surgery, rehab to recover from surgery, or doesn't need surgery at all, our approach is the same. First we make sure the damaged or restricted muscles receive manual treatment. When the muscle damage has sufficiently resolved, we move the patient into the conditioning phase: stretching to restore a normal range of movement, then the strengthening work to build up the resiliency of the treatment area's musculoskeletal system.

THE PROGRAM

We've discussed these ideas in a general way in chapter 1. In this chapter, we're going to distill our strategy into a program the reader can use at home. Our program has the same three parts: muscular self-treatment, stretching, and strength work. It's designed for several different groups of people: for the person with no health problems whatsoever who uses our muscle treatment and conditioning work as a prevention strategy; the person with minor aches and pains who has been cleared by a medical professional to work on these issues on his or her own; someone who's currently being treated by a doctor but who has been cleared to supplement that treatment with our program; and lastly someone who has completed a course of medical treatment and has been cleared to do maintenance work on his or her own. Almost everybody can use it!

But, before we go any further, let's take a closer look at those three areas—treatment, stretching, and strengthening—so you can see how our program evolved.

MANUAL THERAPY TREATMENT

A whole universe of hands-on therapies and therapists exists to treat your muscles. There is no central organization, so seeking out help can be daunting, even though there is no shortage of talented people. What follows are a few of the schools or traditions most accepted by modern medicine. Acupuncture and acupressure target precise spots on the body at which to apply therapeutic pressure, using needles (acupuncture) and manual pressure (acupressure). Chiropractic mobilizes joints and relieves nerve entrapments and muscle spasms. Physical therapy is an umbrella term. Some physical therapists are essentially rehabilitation specialists focusing on muscle conditioning, while others use a range of hands-on techniques. Some individual styles of manual therapy have mostly emerged in the last six decades or so, often blending old and new techniques, and are practiced by health-care professionals from many different disciplines. A few of the most well known are Active Release Techniques (ART), Graston Technique, Myofascial Release, Orthopedic Massage, and Trigger Point Therapy. The granddaddy of hands-on work is therapeutic massage, which has been around in one form or another for centuries.

All of these approaches, from ancient to modern, have their particular methods and their own explanations for how and why they work. Some of them talk about manually breaking up microscopic scar tissue or "adhesions" (ART) or nodules of painfully contracted muscle (Trigger Point Therapy). But broadly considered, they're all trying to do pretty much the same thing: relax tight muscles, relieve pressure on the joints and nerves, and, in most general terms, bring movement (and with it, blood flow and oxygen) to a musculoskeletal system that may have grown restricted and stagnant.

STRETCHING

As discussed, stretching has generated a lot of skepticism in the sports medicine world. Study after study has failed to find much benefit from it: it does not improve athletic performances nor reduce injury rates. But here's the catch. The research has only looked at the traditional "static" form of stretching where you hold the stretch. (Picture a jogger with his leg up on the park bench and bending at the waist, reaching for his toes.)

The stretches we think are most generally valuable are "dynamic." They incorporate movement, and the stretch is never held for more than a couple of seconds, if at all. So is static stretching bad? No. Static stretching has its uses, as do all the stretching styles. Once again, it's a question of matching the right solution with the right problem. Here's a quick and simple look at what's available.

- Static stretching is the conventional and probably still the most popular way to stretch. The static stretcher typically brings the muscle right to the end of its range of motion and holds it there for twenty or thirty seconds. Over time, the muscles, tendons, and ligaments can lengthen, which increases flexibility, but flexible tendons and ligaments are not generally a good thing. Gymnasts, dancers, and martial artists benefit from this improvement in "end range," but most athletes, recreational or elite, play sports that don't need any special flexibility (distance running, cycling, etc.), so for them the argument in favor of static stretching isn't strong. In fact, static stretching, rather than preparing the body for a workout, may weaken the muscle for a time, making it the worst possible pre-workout choice. Furthermore, even if an area of the body has been properly warmed up beforehand, a static stretch can trigger a muscle reflex that actually tightens the muscle, which may lead to irritation of the tendon/muscle area. In postsurgical rehab, static stretching can be effective for breaking down or preventing the formation of scar tissue in order to bring a joint back to a normal range of movement.

- Dynamic stretches incorporate movement, usually emphasizing continuous, rhythmic motion (see the stretch exercises on page 53) that brings blood to the area, loosening and warming up muscles and tendons and preparing them for the increased effort of a workout. They also provide a safe way to relax muscles that have been stressed and shortened during a workout, for example, a run or weight-lifting session. They're equally good for the nonathlete moving through the middle or senior years, as a way to counteract the tightening and stiffening of the connective tissue that occurs with age.

- Active-isolated stretching is a specific type of dynamic stretching (see the stretches at the end of the "hot-spot" chapters). The motion is rhythmic and the stretch is held for no more than two seconds. These stretches provide an effective way to restore a normal range of motion in targeted muscles without stressing tendons or triggering the body reflexes that tighten up muscles.

STRENGTH WORK

The muscles are one of the body's shock absorbers and an important line of defense against damage to the joints. Building up strength in the muscles and connective tissues that stabilize and drive the joints is the goal of the final phase of our strategy and program. We're not interested in pumping up "trophy" muscles in the gym. We want to balance strength in opposing muscle groups (agonist and antagonist) so that the joints have the necessary muscle support throughout their entire range of motion. Every form of strength work comes with built-in advantages and disadvantages. Understand which types of exercises will help you best meet your fitness goals.

- Weight machines in the gym often become the path of least resistance for the novice, but they can be the most limiting form of strength work. The machine controls the movement so only some of the muscles in a movement pattern are used. The machines can be useful, especially for seniors or people with joint dysfunction who may not be able to handle some of the other types of exercises. Working on a range of machines with a knowledgeable personal trainer can be a great start, but you should still try to supplement with other strength exercises.

- Body-weight exercises such as push-ups and core exercises on a stability, or "physio" ball, provide the best foundation for "functional" body strength and balance—what you need to negotiate in the real world. They work a range of muscles from different angles, especially the essential core muscles that stabilize the entire body. Movement-based exercise—for instance, swinging a kettle bell—provides a similar benefit.
- Resistance exercises using a rubber cable, an elastic band, or dumbbells allows you to isolate and develop specific muscles (hopefully after you've achieved a good all-around strength base). Because you have to control the movement of the exercise, unlike with machines, you're also getting some benefit by working supporting neighboring muscles and core muscles.

THE MUSCLE MEDICINE PROGRAM

We've taken from our three-phase strategy what we think are the best techniques for you to do easily and effectively at home. Our stretches are active-isolated, and our strength exercises, a mix of body-weight and resistance work, are basically an at-home version of what you'd get working with a good personal trainer or physical therapist. (We called on one of our favorites, Toni McGinley of Manhattan's Alta Fitness, to help us choose and modify them.) The self-treatment section requires a little more explanation.

A particularly effective self-treatment technique we like to use uniquely modifies concepts from a number of muscle therapies. This unique technique is called F.A.S.T.™, for Facilitated Active Stretch Technique.™ In simplest terms, you are using an external pressure—your fingers, a ball, a stick—to "pin" the muscle near a tight, restricted area. In a conventional stretch, most of the tension builds up at the end of the muscle at its junction with the tendon. When you pin a muscle, you replace the natural endpoint of the stretch with one you define. While maintaining this pin with external pressure, you take the muscle through a range of motion, putting the targeted muscle fibers under tension. This allows you to focus your stretch at the area of tightness or damage. You can effectively control which part of the muscle you stretch, which makes your stretch versatile and therapeutic rather than generalized. (For example, bring the back of your open hand toward your body as if you're signaling "stop" and bend your elbow. With the thumb of the other hand pointing in toward the body, apply pressure down and in on the meaty, top part of the forearm muscle. While maintaining thumb pressure, make a fist and curl it down, then straighten the elbow. You've just done a F.A.S.T.™ stretch to relieve the wrist extensor muscles that can tense up from too many hours at the keyboard.)

We'll give you the precise how-to at the end of the "hot-spot" chapters, but here are the general F.A.S.T.™ principles:

1. By applying pressure at specific spots on the muscle, you pin the muscle just above or below the tight, restricted area.
2. As the muscle is actively taken through a movement, the altered "attachment point" allows you to focus the stretch at the most restricted part of the muscle, where it's most needed. You reach more of the affected fibers.
3. Actively using the antagonist muscles to move the target muscle triggers a reflex that relaxes that muscle. And you're generating physical heat that warms up and loosens the tissues.
4. If you are dealing with an injury, F.A.S.T.™ enables you to target the muscles and connective tissues around it without irritating the compromised tissue. Taking tension off this injured tissue by reducing the pulling forces from the surrounding muscles and connective tissues creates an environment of faster, better healing. Decreased tension on surrounding blood vessels also allows more blood flow to the area, which further promotes healing.

To simplify the job of knowing where to press down, we've provided descriptions with each treatment, dividing the muscle groups we're working on into two or three zones when that's necessary: inner, outer, and, if needed, middle. You start at one end of a zone and move up or down every couple of inches until you've covered the whole region. We'll show you how to apply pressure on the muscle, using "angular" pressure while moving through and completing the movement. You won't be bearing directly down on the muscle but rather angling your force either up or down. More specific directions accompany each muscle treatment in the "hot spot" chapters.

TREATMENT ZONES

We will demonstrate to you exactly where you should be applying angled pressure during treatment. Following the self-treatment instructions, place your hand or treatment tool on the areas described in the figures.

Example: The Infraspinatus.

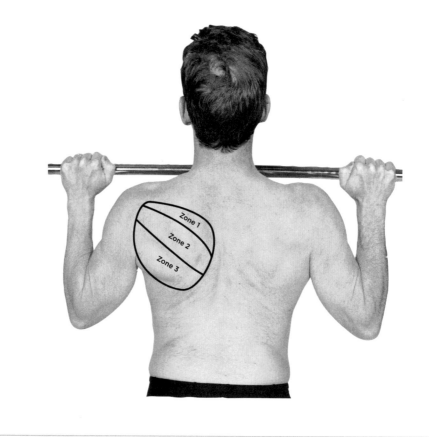

ANGLED PRESSURE

Angled pressure, as introduced in our self-help section in chapers 8–14, is a key part of our self-treatment method. We recommend it whenever you are working with soft tissue. It will help you treat an area of the muscle, tendon, or ligament while controlling your pressure, and help you to work with the muscle fibers. It is performed by first pressing your thumb, fingers, or treatment tool straight into the muscle just deep enough to engage it (Fig. 1), and then by angling the applied force either against or with the movement of the muscle (depending on which direction will generate the tension needed to treat that muscle) (Fig. 2). Keep in mind that there is a learning curve with this. Be patient, as it may take several attempts to feel comfortable with the action.

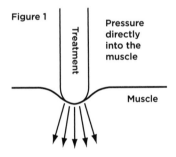

Figure 1

Treatment

Pressure directly into the muscle

Muscle

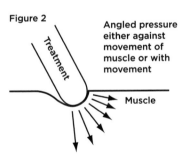

Figure 2

Treatment

Angled pressure either against movement of muscle or with movement

Muscle

We like to describe the self-treatment method as simple but not necessarily easy. Hands-on manual therapy always has a learning curve. As for the muscle medicine program in general, you might consider enlisting the assistance of a physical or muscle therapist to get started and to help you find your own comfort level. New York Giants All-Pro punter Jeff Feagles has. In addition to the world-class athletic training and medical care he receives with the Giants, he's followed our plan, working his hamstrings with F.A.S.T.™, then moving through the dynamic stretches and the strength work that round out the program. During the 2008 season, his punts have soared higher than ever, earning him an invitation to the 2009 NFL Pro Bowl.

INFO

F.A.S.T.™ TREATMENT

Facilitated Active Stretch Technique, or F.A.S.T.™, is a form of dynamic or movement-based stretching that Dr. DeStefano has developed over the years for his patients. Using your hand or a tool such as a F.A.S.T. Stick,™ or other therapeutic stick, apply pressure around a restricted or damaged area, or on a series of points running up and down the muscle, while simultaneously putting the muscle through a range of motion. This allows you to achieve a more effective, precisely targeted stretch. It's a highly effective way to make the structures around an injury relax and to promote healing. You can also use F.A.S.T.™ as part of a regular stretching routine to address muscles used during a workout, such as tight calf muscles after a run or tight biceps after weight lifting.

THE NECK

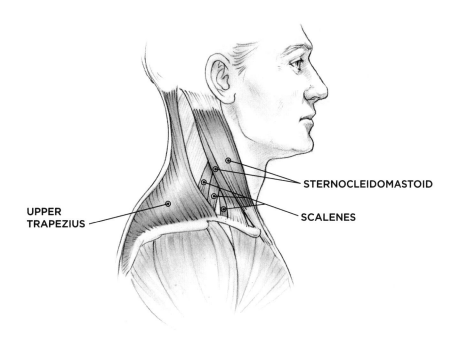

UPPER
TRAPEZIUS

STERNOCLEIDOMASTOID

SCALENES

INTRODUCING THE NECK

There's a reason they call it a "pain in the neck." The bones, ligaments, and muscles that make up the neck have the crucial job of supporting the heavy human head, not only keeping it upright but also allowing it to flex forward, extend backward, and twist from side to side. (Humans evolved as hunters and as the hunted; it pays

THE SPINE

The spine is a vertical stack of twenty-six movable segments that we think of as five distinct sections. Starting from the top, there is the neck or cervical spine, the midback or thoracic spine, the lower back or lumbar spine, and, providing a stabilizing anchor just above the waist, the sacrum. The fifth section, the coccyx or tailbone, is generally not considered structurally important.

The spine evolved to handle two essential jobs: to support the body and to protect the spinal cord. As we move, the spinal column keeps us upright, connecting the upper and lower body in a flexible way so that we can bend and flex and rotate from side to side. That same structure of linked bones or vertebrae doubles as a protective housing for the spinal cord, which passes through it. The spinal cord is a rubbery bundle of millions of nerve fibers—think of a dense fiber-optic cable—that transmits information back and forth between headquarters (the brain) and the branch offices (the peripheral nervous system, which wires the rest of the body). For virtually everything you feel (that would be your sensory neurons firing) and every move you make (your motor neurons firing), data travels up and down the spinal cord as part of an ongoing circular conversation between brain and body.

A lot of craftsmanship has gone into the spinal column. Each vertebra is a cylinder of bone with generally three bony prominences. The side prominences join each vertebra with the one above and below, forming two sets of facet joints, which help guide movement. In between the center of each vertebra are the disks—firm cartilage on the outside, gelatinous on the inside—which act as shock absorbers, contributing to the flexibility of the spine and preventing the bony vertebrae from grinding into each other. Like any hardware, the spine wears down over time. Of all the areas of the spine, the disks can be the most vulnerable pieces.

to have a wide field of vision.) All that movement can cause wear and tear. For that matter, holding your head and neck in a fixed position while staring at a computer screen for hours on end can fatigue the system and invite its own set of pains.

In every "hot-spot" chapter, we want to lay out how the three elements of the system—bone, joint, and muscle—come together to support and drive the human

IMMEDIATE TREATMENT/WHEN TO SEE A DOCTOR

When it comes to possible spinal cord injury, caution rules. If you've suffered a serious blow to the head or neck, see a doctor immediately. You need to rule out damage to the nerves or to the structures of the spinal column, including the vertebrae, the spinal cord, the spinal ligaments, and the disks. Even if there is no obvious trauma, debilitating neck pain or numbness in any part of your body, or shooting pains down your arm, require medical attention right away. If there's any change in bowel or bladder function, get to the emergency room. Any loss of consciousness associated with a neck injury also requires immediate attention. At the least, you may have a concussion. As with any joint problem, look for any signs of infection such as redness and fever or heat. If there are any, see a doctor immediately.

body, and how, when there is pain and dysfunction, they fall out of sync. But the neck (cervical spine) and lower back (lumbar spine) are somewhat special cases. Medical science is good at spotting damage to the bones, ligaments, and disks of the spine on an X-ray and MRI, but so far it doesn't always show the exact connection between damage and actual symptoms.

In fact, the best spine specialists will tell you they don't always know what causes most pain in the cervical and lumbar spine, or why one person has no symptoms and another is in agony when their MRIs show similar amounts of joint damage. Research and experience indicate that this difference can be attributed to muscle. But still we approach the spine with diagnostic humility. In most of the other hot spots we'll be talking about, for instance the hip or the shoulder, we try to be as specific as possible, identifying the individual muscles that act on the joints to cause particular problems. With the neck and the lower back, we're happy to take a "big picture" approach, focusing on a few muscle groups that yield excellent treatment (and self-treatment) results no matter what the textbook definition of the injury is. Those labels (scalene anticus syndrome, for example) are long on anatomical precision and short on clues as to how best to treat the problem. As we'll explain, surgery for cervical and lumbar spine problems is in most cases an option of last resort.

COMMON PROBLEMS AND CULPRITS

The scalene muscles and the sternocleidomastoid muscle in the front of the neck fire to flex the head forward. When they relax, the erector spinae and the suboccipital muscles in the back of the neck engage and extend the head backward. When the neck is flexed forward too far or for too long, the suboccipitals at the base of the skull can tense up, entrapping nerves, which can trigger a tension headache, or "occipital neuralgia." The scalenes can entrap the nerves in the front of the neck, sending pain and numbness down the arm. These symptoms are similar to a more serious case of nerve impingement: when a disk or some part of a bony vertebra presses down on, or "impinges," a nerve root exiting the spinal cord.

WHAT GOES WRONG, AND HOW TO FIX IT

Mostly Muscular

Chronic Neck (Cervical) Strain

John, forty-five, is an accountant in Westchester, New York, who spends the better part of every day slumped over his computer screen poring over the tax returns and balance sheets of his corporate clients. During tax season, he'll stay mostly glued to the spot for eight to twelve hours at a stretch, take-out lunch containers and empty cans of Diet Coke piling up beside his work files. For years, his wife has been after him about his poor posture—his shoulders are rounded and his neck and head project forward instead of being in line with the rest of his spine. He ignored her until he started to be bothered by a laundry list of aches and pains that interfered with his productivity at work. His neck seems perpetually achy and sore, his shoulder throbs in the vicinity of his shoulder blade, and he's starting to get "tension headaches" that attack the top of his scalp.

Imagine holding a bowling ball, which weighs about as much as a human head, up over your head. Hold it directly overhead, in line with your spine, and it's not so bad. You can maintain the pose for a while. But let your arms fall forward, and the effort quickly becomes excruciating as you stress the arm muscles and the supporting muscles of the chest and back. That's what it's like for your neck when your head is not in line, and why good posture is important.

As John painfully discovered, the spine can only handle the forces of gravity without irritation when it's in balance. That doesn't mean straight up and down, otherwise nature would have equipped us with a solid rod for a backbone (not much flexibility or shock absorption there). Instead our spinal column is a stack of four gently curving C-shaped segments that balance and counterbalance each other: the cervical spine curves forward, the thoracic spine curves backward, the lumbar spine forward, and the sacrum backward. This design functions as a spring. The soft tissues hold this graceful sculpture in place, and a network of ligaments run up and down the spine like supporting ropes. Opposing muscles in front and back of the spine do their part to provide balanced, flexible support.

When John's shoulders slump forward and his neck and head settle into this forward position, he's overstretching some of the muscles in the front of his neck and upper back and overworking muscles in the front, sides, and back of the neck, shoulders, and upper back. The result is pain of at least a couple of different kinds. As we described in chapter 3, the overworked muscles can contract so forcefully as to cause pain directly. Or muscles in the neck can spasm and entrap nerves running down into the shoulder. John has pain in both areas. (The neck/shoulder connection is a close and often uncomfortable one.) The neck-forward position strains the suboccipital muscles at the base and sides of the skull, which can entrap nerves that run up the back of the head, causing John's tension headaches. (A couple of John's colleagues who haven't made the switch to telephone headsets have one more muscular affliction: achy muscles from cradling a receiver between a hunched shoulder and a sideways-bent neck.)

Skeletally, nothing is seriously wrong with John. Muscularly, he is a mess. And if he does nothing to address his slumpy sitting posture at work, the loss of the normal curve in the cervical spine may finally put enough pressure on the disks to seriously damage them, in which case all the pain and suffering he's endured to this point will only have been a warm-up act.

The conventional medical approach to John's problems could be to put him on an over-the-counter anti-inflammatory such as Advil (ibuprofen) and be done with it. These drugs effectively dull pain, which can help the body to relax and a person to get back to life, but they don't treat the root of the problem, which still exists when the drugs wear off. More powerful prescription muscle-relaxant drugs are also an option, but they have the same pros and cons. The sensible approach would be to benefit from the anti-inflammatories while pursuing a course of treatment that addresses the underlying issue. John should improve his ergonomics and work habits (see the box on page 86) and go to physical therapy. The therapist will most likely work on bringing his head and neck back in line with the rest of the spine with conditioning exercises that stretch out the tight muscles of the neck and chest, and then strengthen the muscles in his neck and upper back.

But there's another angle to this story. Slumpers may be born as well as made. John may have a genetic predisposition to age into that rounded-shoulder posture, and it's certain that the years of working hunched over his keyboard have retrained his brain-muscle connection, his "proprioceptive" sense of where his body should be, so that slumping has come to feel normal. Four or so sessions of insurance-covered PT isn't going to change that. Moreover, jumping into strength and stretching exercises when his muscles are still contracted and inflamed is likely to do more harm than good.

Timing is everything. The ideal first-line treatment is manual therapy that relieves pain by relaxing muscle tension, especially in the scalenes, which pull the neck forward as they tighten up. When he's pliable enough, he can get some real benefit from physical therapy, which is necessary for muscular reeducation. In the best of all worlds, John will incorporate some of his PT exercises into his everyday routine, using them to counter the forces of gravity and bad work habits. (You'll be introduced to muscular self-treatment techniques, stretching, and strength-conditioning exercises at the end of this chapter.) Will John's commitment to reeducate his body give him perfect posture? Probably not, but it may be enough to keep him out of pain and spare his disks serious damage. Even if all he takes away from PT is the habit of checking in with his body once or twice a day to relax the shoulders and let them drop, that could be enough.

Geri is a corporate road warrior who logs countless miles on the road and, back at the home office, too many hours sitting in meetings in uncomfortable office chairs.

She's got the spine of a warrior too. Her MRI reveals that a couple of the disks in her cervical spine are starting to deteriorate—a combination of normal aging and the demands of her hard-charging lifestyle. That makes her more vulnerable to the contracted muscles and pain in her neck and shoulders that Dr. DeStefano has successfully treated off and on with manual therapy for five years. But when she came into his office recently, she could barely move her head. She'd just completed a big business deal, and the stress and constant air travel had triggered a major flare-up of symptoms. Dr. DeStefano worked on the scalenes and longissimus colli on the front of the neck and performed some gentle chiropractic adjustments. After two treatments Geri was ready to return to battle.

As you age, the jellylike material that fills the inside of the vertebral disks loses water, shrinks, and hardens, which is one reason you lose height in the middle and senior years. (The disks account for a full 20 percent of your height.) The disks become less flexible and less adept at absorbing shock, which in turn can make the firm cartilage material that forms the outer layer of the disks more prone to cracking. This doesn't mean you're doomed to neck and back pain as you get older. But it does mean that as you subject your spine to the usual use and abuse of living, the margin of error gets smaller.

Geri's case is typical. It's possible that worn disks contributed to her pain. The nerves around the disks may have gotten irritated and sent distress signals to the muscles, which shut down as a protective measure. We don't know. But we're reasonably sure from diagnostic tests and from the on-and-off nature of her pain that the muscles are the primary issue. It just took a couple of stressful weeks of work to send them over the edge into painful dysfunction. Remember the process we described in chapter 4. Psychological stress caused her to unconsciously tense the muscles in her neck and shoulders, further reducing the supply of oxygen to the area, and to breathe more shallowly. The considerable time she logged in airline seats, with inadequate support for her neck and lower back, finished the job. (See the box on page 86 on how to minimize wear and tear on the road.) The solution was to bring movement back to her muscles and joints by treating them manually and to coach her on some deep-breathing exercises.

PROTECT YOUR NECK

Don't tilt your head down when you read. If you wear reading glasses, don't pull your head back to get the proper focus. Don't adjust your head position to the material, adjust the material to you. Try to keep your head in a neutral position.

When you watch TV at home, make sure that your couch or chair is directly facing the TV and that your neck is adequately supported, for instance, with a pillow.

When you're traveling by plane or train, bring a small pillow for better neck support.

Don't sleep on your stomach. If you must, alternate the side you turn your neck to. Your pillow should support your head and keep it in line with the spine.

Don't bend your neck down to look at the keyboard when you type. (In other words, don't "hunt and peck.")

Set up your computer monitor so you can look at it dead-on without tilting your head up or down.

If you spend a lot of time on the phone, invest in a headset. Do not cradle the phone receiver between your ear and your shoulder.

Take frequent, short work breaks. Move around to get the blood flowing in your upper body. A quick exercise, such as rolling your shoulders, is great.

Traumatic Neck Strain (Whiplash)

While he was a running back, Tiki Barber woke up one Monday morning so battered by Sunday night's game that he had to use his hand to help raise his head off the pillow. He'd figured he'd done something serious like broken his shoulder blade. After being examined and cleared by the medical staff, he received daily treatment from the athletic trainers. Part of his treatment included work with Dr. DeStefano, who released his tight, contracted muscles and administered chiropractic adjustments. Barber was able to return to play the very next Sunday.

If injury is chronic (i.e., from twenty years spent hunched over a computer keyboard) or acute (from one violent instant on the football field), damage to muscle creates scar tissue, and a manual therapist will treat it much the same way. But when the head and neck snap back in a "whiplash" injury (think rear-end car collision), both muscles and ligaments are subjected to tremendous pressure. Because ligaments heal so poorly and because they are crucial for neck support, a ligament tear in the cervical spine is serious business and can result in permanent weakness and instability. Tiki Barber's problem, fortunately, was mostly muscular. As Barber discovered, it's amazing how incapacitating "only" a muscle problem can be, and how quickly, with the right treatment, the tissue can bounce back.

Muscle or Joint?

Cervical Disk Pain

Barbara, a forty-three-year-old Manhattan banker, suffered from persistent neck pain. Not only had the discomfort gotten worse in recent weeks, but she was experiencing shooting pains down her arm. The MRI showed that two of her disks were damaged and could be part of the problem. But Dr. DeStefano felt that if he could get the neck muscles to relax, he could probably bring her out of the pain. He worked on her and achieved some improvement but not enough. That suggested that the damaged disks and not the muscles were the primary culprit. He sent Barbara to Dr. Jennifer Solomon, a physiatrist at Manhattan's Hospital for Special Surgery who specializes in the spine and sports medicine. She gave Barbara an injection of a corticosteroid anti-inflammatory near the disk, which immediately cut the pain by 90 percent. Barbara then received more manual treatment on the irritated muscles before moving on to physical therapy, where she worked on improving her posture and stretching and strengthening her neck muscles. Four months after she first walked into Dr. DeStefano's office, her neck and arm pain were gone and life had returned to normal.

When a disk herniates, the outer, firm cartilage tears and some of the inner pulp leaks out. (The old popular term for this was *slipped disk,* which paints the wrong picture.) The innards can irritate the surrounding nerves physically, by pressing against them, or the nerves can be irritated chemically, by inflammatory proteins surrounding the injury. One solution is to surgically remove the damaged disk and fuse the two, now diskless, vertebrae together. But even the surgeons who perform this delicate surgery consider it a last resort after all less invasive measures have failed.

Considering the state of Barbara's cervical disks, it's logical to conclude that they were causing the radiating arm pain. Logical but not always right. Studies show that one in five people under the age of sixty with no spine pain have herniated disks. It's quite possible to have disk damage that isn't the direct or most important cause of your neck or lower-back pain. The muscles in the neck, the scalenes in particular, can become inflamed and irritate the surrounding nerves, causing those disturbing symptoms of pain, numbness, or tingling. The medical establishment has an impressive-sounding diagnostic label for the condition, *scalene anticus syndrome,* but its focus is often drug therapy.

In our experience, the best approach to these kinds of spinal problems is the most conservative one. If muscle therapy doesn't solve the problem, it should point us in the right diagnostic direction. As it turned out, Barbara's herniated disks were impinging on the nerves, causing the muscles to shut down, which only compounded the problem. A team approach—medical treatment (the steroid injection), muscle therapy, and physical therapy—resolved the case without surgery. Research shows that most of these herniated-disk problems in the cervical (and lumbar) spine do not need surgery. Often the pain clears up on its own in months for reasons no one yet understands. Dr. Solomon, who consults with both of us on some of our toughest cases, surgical and manual, has had good success with a single corticosteroid injection that can immediately quiet the nerve irritation. By breaking the cycle of pain and inflammation even temporarily, we give the body a fighting chance to begin to heal on its own.

Joint/Orthopedic

Cervical Disk Pain (with Severe Neurological Symptoms)
If the nerve pain that radiates down through the body is severe and unrelenting, and the muscles connected to those nerves are getting progressively weaker, medical attention is crucial and surgery may be your best option.

Osteoarthritis
You may not think of a neck as being arthritic in the same way you might a knee or a hip. But the joints that hold the vertebrae together do often wear out. When that happens, vertebra rubs against vertebra, bone against bone, and pain and possibly arthritis can result.

We can't say for sure how much of the pain is being generated by the damaged spine itself and how much by the surrounding muscles that tighten up in response to the injury signals sent from the spine. Since no one knows how to stop arthritis in its tracks directly, manual therapy—which relaxes the muscles in the

INFO

WHAT IS A PHYSIATRIST?

A physiatrist is an M.D. who specializes in the diagnosis and treatment of muscle and joint problems, including rehabilitation, physical medicine, and pain management. If you have chronic neck or lower-back pain, you may consider getting the opinion of a physiatrist in addition to that of an orthopedist.

neck, providing at least some symptomatic pain relief—can be an important part of the "toolbox." Anti-inflammatory drugs and occasional corticosteroid injections have their place. But the person living with arthritis needs to make important adjustments to put less stress on the spinal architecture: lose weight; get on a low-impact exercise program; do physical therapy to improve posture. "You have to look at the whole picture," Dr. Solomon says. "And having the patient take control is really important."

INFO

WHEN SURGERY IS THE BEST OPTION

There are certain spine issues that are clearly surgical cases:

1. Disk herniations with loss of motor control or strength deficit
2. Disk herniations with loss of bowel or bladder continence
3. Spinal stenosis with motor symptoms or neurogenic claudication (weakness and/or painful cramping stemming from the nerve)

Spinal Stenosis

Spinal stenosis can develop anywhere along the spine. When the vertebrae develop bone spurs or the disks protrude, for instance, the space inside the spinal column narrows, compressing the nerves that run through it. Pain, numbness, and weakness in the arms, hands, or legs can be the unhappy result.

Older patients can often be poor candidates for surgery. For them, and many other patients, a combination of manual and physical therapy and, when needed, corticosteroid injections, is a very effective approach to relieving symptoms. However, decompression surgeries of nerves entrapped due to stenosis directly address the cause of the symptoms and are probably some of the most effective and predictable spine surgeries.

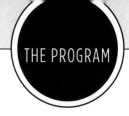

NECK

We divide the neck into three treatment areas: the front, back, and sides (anterior, posterior, and lateral). The movements include flexion (bringing the chin to the chest), extension (chin to the ceiling), lateral flexion (ear to shoulder), rotation (chin toward shoulder), and some coupled movements (a combination of the previous movements). The neck has so many possibilities of movement because it is designed to aid the eyes in taking in as full a scope of vision as possible. Contact your health-care professional if numbness or tingling occurs in the upper extremities during any of the following self-treatment, stretches, or exercises.

ANTERIOR (FRONT) NECK MUSCLES

A. SCALENES

Purpose: To target and remove restrictions and restore a full range of motion to the anterior neck muscles (especially the scalenes) by manually releasing tight, short, and damaged muscles.

Starting out: Sit on a stability ball or chair with your feet spread shoulders' width apart. Flex your neck and tuck your chin. Hold your index and middle fingers together and place them on the front of the neck between your Adam's apple and ear line. Your fingers should rest behind the large muscle running diagonally across the neck, the sternocleidomastoid (SCM).

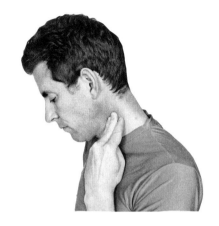

How to do it: Press in and down slightly, as though trying to prevent someone from sliding a sheet of paper from under your fingers. Tilt your head back, look up, and extend the neck. Hold for a count of two. Repeat on the opposite side. Do two to three repetitions, releasing and moving your hand position from higher to lower each time.

Troubleshooting: Don't press too hard as this can irritate the muscles. Avoid putting too much pressure over the blood vessels of the neck. Avoid letting your skin slide under your fingers by using angled pressure. (See the "Angled Pressure" box on page 77.) Keep the stretch gentle—do not strain the muscle.

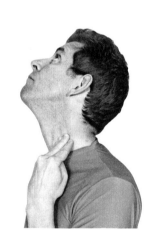

*Important: Check with your doctor before attempting any work on your anterior neck, especially if you suffer from cardiovascular disease or "hardening" of the arteries (atherosclerosis).

B. STERNOCLEIDOMASTOID

Purpose: To target and remove restrictions and restore a full range of motion to the anterior neck muscles (especially the SCM) by manually releasing tight, short, and damaged muscles.

Starting out: Sit on a stability ball or chair with your feet spread shoulders' width apart. Turn from the chin and look down toward the opposite knee. Using the hand opposite to the treatment side, hold your index and middle fingers together and place them on the front of the neck between your Adam's apple and ear line. Your fingers should rest on the big muscle of the neck (SCM).

How to do it: Press in and down slightly, as though trying to prevent someone from sliding a sheet of paper from under your fingers. Turn the head toward the treatment side, looking up and past the treatment-side shoulder. There should be a stretch on the front of the neck, but not too much tension in the back. Hold for a count of two each time. Repeat on the opposite side. Do two to three repetitions, moving your hand position from the top of the muscle down toward the base.

Troubleshooting: Don't press too hard as this can irritate the muscle. Avoid putting too much pressure over the blood vessels of the neck. Avoid letting the skin slide under the fingers by using angled pressure.

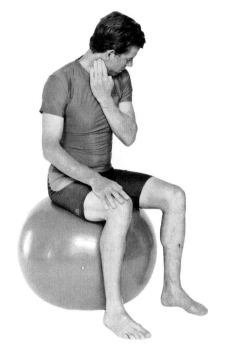

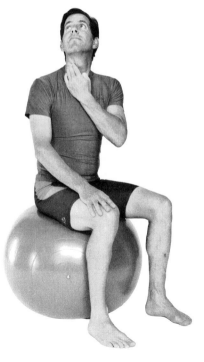

POSTERIOR (BACK) NECK MUSCLES

Purpose: To target and remove any restrictions and restore a full range of motion to the posterior neck muscles (cervical erector spinae, upper trapezius, and deep intrinsic muscles) by manually releasing tight, short, and damaged muscles. This is a real hot spot for anyone who works at a computer, studies, or suffers from headaches.

Starting out: Sit on a stability ball or chair with your feet spread shoulders' width apart. Keeping an upright posture, tilt your head back. Hold your index, middle, and ring fingers together and place the fingertips on the back of the neck. Find the spine and then move over about an inch onto the thick muscle.

How to do it: Press in and down slightly so that the fingers don't slide with the movement. Bring your head forward as though trying to gently hold a tennis ball under the chin. This should be a gentle movement held for a count of two. Repeat on the opposite side. Do two to three repetitions, releasing and moving your hand position from the top to the bottom of the neck each time.

Troubleshooting: Avoid pressing too hard as this can irritate the muscles. Avoid letting the skin slide under the fingers by using angled pressure. Don't collapse the neck back or forward, as it compresses the spine: keep an upright posture.

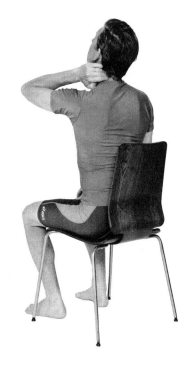

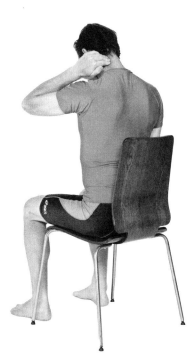

LATERAL (SIDE) NECK MUSCLES

Purpose: To target and remove any restrictions and restore a full range of motion to side (lateral) muscles, especially in the upper trapezius by manually releasing tight, short, and damaged muscles of the lateral neck. These muscles are also a hot spot for those who spend their days in front of a computer or engage in manual labor.

Starting out: Sit on a stability ball or chair with your feet spread shoulders' width apart. Without letting your head bend forward or back, bring the treatment-side ear toward your shoulder. Find the bony bump behind the ear, bring your fingers behind it, and follow a line down to the base of the neck. Using the hand opposite to the treatment side, hold your index, middle, and ring fingers together and place the finger pads on the target area at the base of the lateral neck.

Apply tension to these three areas: the top of the muscle, especially at the base of the neck; just in front of that muscle; and just behind that muscle.

How to do it: Press in and toward the shoulder slightly so that the fingers stay with the muscle and don't slide. Bring the ear toward the opposite shoulder. Hold for a count of two. Repeat on the opposite side. Do two to three repetitions on three points per zone, moving from the neck out toward the shoulder.

Troubleshooting: Avoid pressing too hard; let the fingers move over the skin and muscle by using angled pressure. The ear should end up over the opposite shoulder; don't let the head drop forward or back or rotate left or right at any point in the movement. Finally, don't lift the shoulder up toward the ear; relax and let the shoulders drop down.

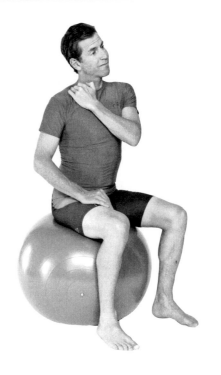

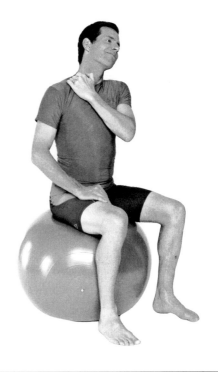

ANTERIOR AND POSTERIOR NECK

Purpose: To bring the muscles of the front and back neck through their pain-free range of motion and warm up the muscles of the neck and upper back.

Starting out: Sit on a stability ball or chair with your feet spread shoulders' width apart. Keeping an upright posture, your head should be neutral with your eyes facing forward.

How to do it: Gently tilt your head forward toward the chest as though gently holding a tennis ball under the chin. Hold for two seconds. Keeping an upright posture, bring the head gently back to the starting position, then tilt the head back, reaching the nose up toward the ceiling. Hold each end position for a count of two. Do ten repetitions, held for no more than two seconds each.

Troubleshooting: Do not let your head collapse forward or back or let your shoulders come up. Keep an upright posture to avoid compression of the neck. You should feel a stretch in the back of your neck, then the front, but not too much tension on the nonstretching side. This should be a gentle movement.

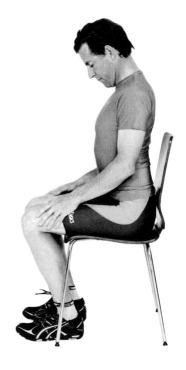

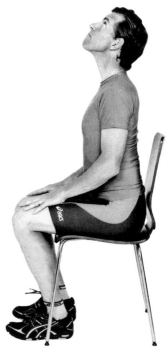

LATERAL NECK

A. LATERAL FLEXION

Purpose: To bring the neck muscles through their pain-free range of motion (ROM). This will warm them up and allow the ends of the ROM to be safely explored.

Starting out: Sit on a stability ball or chair with your feet spread shoulders' width apart. Keeping the head in line with the shoulders, sit up straight.

How to do it: Tilt your head/ear toward one shoulder. If this can be accomplished without pain or compression of the neck, at the end of the movement you can use your hand to gently bring the head a little farther toward the shoulder. Hold for a count of two. Repeat on the opposite side. Do ten repetitions, held for no more than two seconds each.

Troubleshooting: Keep your head in line with your shoulders: don't let it tilt forward or back or rotate left or right at any point in the movement. Don't shrug the shoulders up toward the ears or look to the side—keep looking straight ahead.

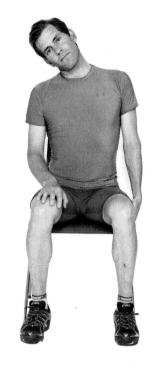

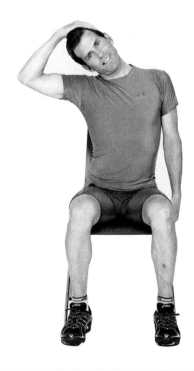

B. ROTATION

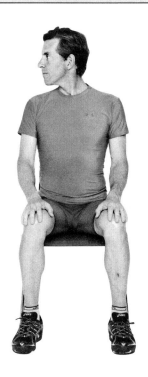

Purpose: To bring the rotational neck muscles through their pain-free range of motion and warm up the muscles of the neck and upper back.

Starting out: Sit on a stability ball or chair with your feet spread shoulders' width apart. The spine should be upright and the eyes facing forward.

How to do it: Rotate the head/chin to the right. Keep the head up to avoid compression of the neck. Hold for a count of two. Repeat on the opposite side. Do ten repetitions, held for no more than two seconds each.

Troubleshooting: This is a gentle movement. There should not be any pain or strain. Do not overtwist the neck, and maintain an upright posture. Avoid flexing your head forward or extending it back.

ALL NECK MUSCLES, SUPERFICIAL TO DEEP
CERVICAL TRACTION WITH TOWEL ROLL

Purpose: This stretch is unique to this book in that it is a passive relaxation (also known as positional release). The deepest musculature is targeted as well as the more superficial layers. Its purpose is to bring the neck muscles into a neutral state and to promote relaxation, especially of tight, spasmed, or imbalanced muscles.

Starting out: Lie on your back with your knees bent and feet flat on the floor. Place a rolled towel under your neck, creating a subtle traction. The spine should be in a neutral position, anatomical curve.

How to do it: The towel roll is a small towel rolled into a cylinder so that it supports the neck comfortably without propping the head off the floor. You should experience comfortable lengthening or "opening" of the neck and a relaxation of all the muscles. (Optionally, you can place a gel ice pack over the towel and cover it with a layer or two of paper towels. Ice for five to fifteen minutes. Repeat after an hour, if necessary.)

Troubleshooting: Stop immediately if there is pain or if symptoms worsen. Don't use too big or too small of a towel roll or the neck will not be neutral and the muscles won't be able to relax completely. The neck should not feel compressed in the front or back. Contact a health-care professional if numbness or tingling occurs in the arms during this or any of the stretches or self-treatment.

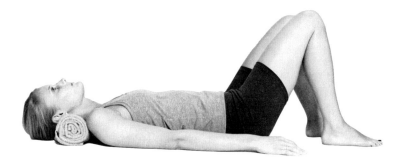

ANTERIOR, POSTERIOR, AND LATERAL NECK

A. HEAD PUSHES AGAINST A WALL

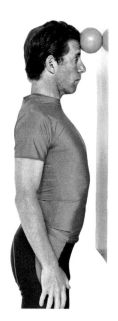

Purpose: To strengthen the muscles of the anterior, posterior, and lateral neck. This will warm them up and increase cervical spine stabilization, which contributes significantly to spine health.

Starting out: (This describes the anterior neck exercise, but the same exercise can be adapted for the back or the sides of the neck.) Stand with your feet shoulders' width apart. Keeping an upright posture and looking forward, place a ball between your head and the wall.

How to do it: Without leaning, press the head gently into the ball, then release. Do ten repetitions, held for no more than two seconds each.

Troubleshooting: Do not push the ball with any significant force. Do not lean the body into the ball. Keep up good posture—do not bend the neck in any other direction while pressing the ball.

B. HEAD PUSHES AGAINST HAND RESISTANCE

Purpose: To strengthen the muscles of the anterior, posterior, and lateral neck. This will warm them up and increase cervical spine stabilization.

Starting out: (This describes the anterior neck exercise, but the same exercise can be adapted for the back or the sides of the neck.) Stand or sit on a stability ball with your feet shoulders' width apart. Keeping an upright posture and looking forward, place a hand on the forehead or the back of the head, or just above the ear on the side of the head.

How to do it: Without leaning, press your head gently into your hand, then release. Do ten repetitions, held for no more than two seconds each.

Troubleshooting: Do not push with any significant force. Do not lean your body into your hand—maintain good posture. Do not bend the neck in any direction while pressing your head into your hand.

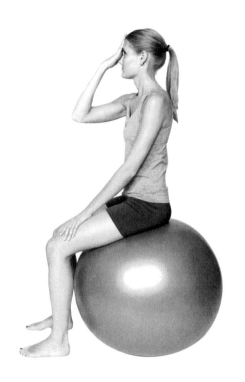

THE SHOULDER

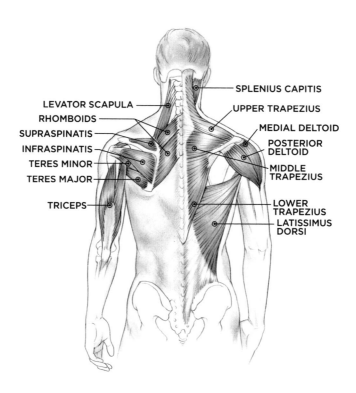

SPLENIUS CAPITIS

LEVATOR SCAPULA

UPPER TRAPEZIUS

RHOMBOIDS

SUPRASPINATIS

MEDIAL DELTOID

INFRASPINATIS

POSTERIOR DELTOID

TERES MINOR

MIDDLE TRAPEZIUS

TERES MAJOR

TRICEPS

LOWER TRAPEZIUS

LATISSIMUS DORSI

INTRODUCING THE SHOULDER

Every joint represents a trade-off between stability and mobility. With the shoulder joint, evolution decided to go for broke and bet everything on mobility. The shoulder can easily move in every direction; its versatility is the reason you can slam a tennis serve or put your clothes on in the morning. The complex movement of the

IMMEDIATE TREATMENT/
WHEN TO SEE A DOCTOR

If you suspect you have a broken bone, see a doctor. Likewise, if the shoulder is dislocated (the humeral head comes out of the socket), even if the shoulder pops back in, with or without assistance. There could be damage to the cartilage, blood vessels, or nerves. If you take a fall and can't move your arm, nerve damage or a tendon rupture are possibilities; either needs to be medically addressed. As with any joint problem, look for any signs of infection—redness, heat or fever, or pain not connected to changes in activity. If there are any, see a doctor immediately. When the dire possibilities have been ruled out, you can assume you've got some kind of soft-tissue damage, usually a muscle or joint strain or sprain. The normal rules of RICE apply: Rest (keep weight off the area); Ice it; keep inflammation down with Compression (for instance, a compression bandage); and Elevation (bring the affected area above the level of your heart). It's your call whether to seek out a doctor or muscle therapist right away, but if pain persists after one or two weeks, it's time.

shoulder is achieved through an elaborate architecture that involves the eighteen muscles and three major bones: the upper-arm bone (humerus), the collarbone (clavicle), and the shoulder blade (scapula). Raising your arm overhead is achieved by a movement of all three bones coordinated by the muscles.

The price for all this freedom of movement is instability. The shoulder joint has a greater propensity to dislocate than all of the body's other joints. Unlike the hip, where the joint seems so solid, the shoulder is such a delicate balancing act you can't help but see how the three elements of the system—bone, joint, muscle—fit together to make the joint work. Take the innermost shoulder joint, technically the glenohumeral joint. The rounded knob of the humerus fits into the shoulder socket at the end of the shoulder blade like a golf ball on a tee. Not exactly a tight fit. It glides and rotates without falling out thanks to a supporting weave of connective tissue and muscle. The foundation of this weave is the rotator cuff. It is the broad, cufflike, common tendinous attachment of four muscles surrounding the shoulder joint. These tendons and their muscles help to coordinate the multiple planes of movement of the shoulder and keep the joint in its place.

COMMON PROBLEMS AND CULPRITS

The eighteen muscles that cross the shoulder offer up lots of good examples of "referred pain," where the source of muscle pain and the location of that pain are in different places. Consider the deltoid muscle, which covers the shoulder on three sides or the sheetlike latissimus dorsi, which wraps from the front of the shoulder down around to the back. Pain is often felt in these large muscles lying just below the skin—therapists will work them, M.D.'s will inject them—but the actual damage can be in the deeper stabilizing muscles, which overwork to keep the shoulder girdle in proper position. The most common of these are the four muscles that form the rotator cuff, whose job it is to keep the shoulder ball properly moving in the socket: the subscapularis, supraspinatus, infraspinatus, and teres minor.

Another muscle often involved in shoulder dysfunction may surprise you because it's so well-known. Even though the biceps sits over the arm, the muscle's two upper heads attach to the shoulder, not the upper-arm bone (the humerus). The biceps is responsible for a lot of heavy lifting and can tighten up, pulling the shoulder blade forward and causing shoulder pain. The more serious cases we label bicipital tendinitis. The tendon attaching the longer of the two biceps heads to the shoulder blade can become so irritated and weakened that it ruptures. Sometimes surgery is the best option.

The upper trapezius muscle is the "shoulder shrugging" muscle of the upper back. This muscle tends to be misused and contracted in a lot of people, contributing to poor posture, and often causing strain and referring pain up to the muscles of the neck (one reason why neck and shoulder pain so often go together).

To stabilize the shoulder girdle, many muscles that attach to the scapula anchor themselves all the way from the skull down to the neck and into the upper back. Shoulder nerves can get impinged by any of these tight muscles and get pulled and irritated. This is another reason shoulder pain is often accompanied by head, neck, and upper-back pain.

PROTECT YOUR SHOULDERS

When you're under stress, notice if you're hunching your shoulders. During the day, make a conscious effort to let them drop.

Use both straps of a backpack to carry your personal gear and work materials, to equalize the pressure on the shoulders. If that's not possible, make a conscious effort to switch shoulders when you carry a shoulder bag.

Don't rub a sore shoulder. It may give temporary relief, but you're only contributing to the inflammation and more pain later. Have a pro who can differentiate between therapy and irritation do it.

The rotator cuff is prone to tearing during extreme activity. In middle age, the most common rotator-cuff injuries come from the wear and tear of repetitive motion. Major tears need to be surgically repaired, whereas some tears can be rehabilitated with a combination of stretching tight muscles and strengthening weak ones.

WHAT GOES WRONG, AND HOW TO FIX IT

Mostly Muscular

Shoulder Strain, or "Rotator-Cuff Strain"

Mary, retired and widowed at seventy-eight, was still in wonderful physical condition and enjoyed her active life. One day, she was standing on top of her kitchen counter changing some curtains when she slipped and fell, banging her arm and shoulder on a tabletop on the way down. The pain in her shoulder took her to her doctor, who was relieved to see on the MRI that she had not torn her rotator cuff. The MRI did show evidence of bursitis (inflammation of the bursa sac), common in the shoulders of older people, and he told her she was just going to have to live with the discomfort. That didn't sit well with Mary, who could no longer put her sweater on without help. When Dr. DeStefano treated her, he found that both her rotator-cuff muscles and her deltoids had been hurt in the fall. The damaged muscles had contracted and created microscopic scar tissue which had bound the muscles to each other. When Mary tried to lift her arm, she was painfully tugging at the muscle tissue. Dr. DeStefano manually broke up the scar tissue, relaxed the muscles, and got them to separate from each other. Mary returned to her normal pain-free life.

When you lose your balance, the natural impulse is to try to break a fall with your outstretched arms. You can thus easily give the shoulder muscles a sudden, traumatic jolt. In Mary's case, because she hadn't torn the rotator-cuff tendons, the muscle damage didn't show up on the MRI. Her doctor blamed her pain on the damage that was visible—the inflammation of the shoulder bursa, or bursitis. But actually her scarred shoulder muscles were painfully disrupting the movement of the entire joint. The mild bursitis hadn't caused her problems before the fall and has yet to cause her problems after. At times the bursa may be the cause of pain, but it is often falsely accused because it is the only visible structural problem.

Becky is a talented seventeen-year-old softball pitcher who plays in one of the highly competitive girls fast-pitch leagues in New Jersey. Last year, her season looked to be over before it had begun. Every time she pitched with her usual velocity, she'd be stopped by pain in her throwing arm. Her orthopedist didn't see any muscle tears on the MRI, only minor inflammation, so he told her to take some time off and sent her to PT to work on muscle strength and conditioning. When she returned to the mound, the pain returned to the shoulder. A couple of rounds of anti-inflammatory injections had only a minor effect. When Dr. DeStefano treated her, he found that a number of her shoulder muscles were misfiring. The big offenders were the rotator-cuff muscles, especially the subscapularis. Traumatized by the repeated force of Becky's pitching motion, it was shortened, tight, and injured, throwing off the movement of the humeral head in the joint and inflaming the entire area. After Dr. DeStefano manually broke up the muscle tightness and the inflammation subsided, she was ready for physical therapy to strengthen her shoulder. Becky was back on her softball team in weeks.

The vulnerable shoulder has a hard time with sports. The pitching motion is particularly tough. The rotator-cuff muscles have to fire strongly, especially to deaccelerate the arm after the pitch is thrown.

The supraspinatus is the "star" of the rotator-cuff group and, being relatively easy to get at on top of the shoulder blade, it gets its share of therapeutic attention. But sometimes the subscapularis is the hidden villain. Located on the underside of the shoulder blade next to the rib cage, when it tightens up, it rotates the arm inwardly. Becky was fighting against her damaged subscapularis every time she went into her pitching motion.

Shoulder Instability

Laura, a teenager from Sheepshead Bay, Brooklyn, New York, swims on the U.S. national team. She was diagnosed with a lax shoulder capsule, fairly common in swimmers. The ligaments that form the capsule that holds the shoulder joint in place were naturally loose. These hypermobile joints can be an advantage in competitive swimming—Michael Phelps is a great example—but for a lot of swimmers they can lead to muscle pain, even shoulder subluxations (partial dislocations). Laura's rotator-cuff muscles were having to overwork to keep the joint in place, and her subscapularis muscle in particular was tight and fatigued. Dr. DeStefano treated her manually to reset the balance of the rotator-cuff muscle group. The tighter muscles were loosened manually. The muscles that had lost strength from being underused were built up in physical therapy.

Like a lot of athletes, when Laura doesn't feel right, she wants to do something to get at the problem. When she felt tightness in her shoulder muscles, she would stretch the area nonstop, further loosening the shoulder capsule, which was the cause of the muscle tightness in the first place. She incessantly rubbed the area as well, and her unskilled direct pressure became another source of muscular irritation. We gave her some stretches and strength exercises that targeted the correct muscles (see the program of self-treatment and stretches at the end of the chapter), and she happily returned to the national swim team.

Muscle or Joint?

Rotator-Cuff Tendinitis/Partial Tears

For most of us, rotator-cuff injury is a story of slow decline. With age, the tendons lose their suppleness. They become irritated rubbing against the bony underside of the shoulder blade when the arm lifts up into the overhead position. Painful tendinitis sets in and the rotator-cuff muscles begin to shut down, throwing off the motion of the shoulder ball in the socket. The ball can ride too high, pushing the cuff tendons against the tip of the shoulder blade (impingement), compounding the damage. (The bony tip itself may be shaped in such way as to gouge the cuff tendons.) Usually the best way to stop the downward spiral is manual therapy to address the muscles and, when the inflammation and irritation have calmed down, physical therapy to build up strength in the rotator cuff and surrounding muscles. Otherwise, tendinitis can so weaken the tissue, the tendon tears, partially or completely. Partial tears can heal by themselves, "full thickness" tears cannot and often require surgery.

Frozen Shoulder (Adhesive Capsulitis)

Busy with family and volunteer work, Joan had let her tennis game go for the past few years. When she moved to a new neighborhood and discovered the nice public courts, she threw herself into a regular schedule of twice-a-week tennis, good exercise for a woman now in her early fifties. She didn't make any extra time for conditioning or stretching, but that didn't seem to affect her game. Several weeks into her new routine she began waking up at night with a dull ache in her shoulder. She had to experiment with comfortable positions just to get back to sleep. The pain became sharper, disturbing her days as well as her nights, and she was losing range of motion in her shoulder. Putting a coat on became difficult, so you can guess what playing tennis felt like. Her orthopedist diagnosed "frozen shoulder"—the fibrocartilage capsule that encases the shoulder joint was shrinking and tightening, causing the pain and restricted movement. He explained that surgery is rarely the best option and sent her to a physical therapist to strengthen the shoulder. Fortunately the therapist was well versed in manual techniques. Before launching into the strengthening exercises that would overload the damaged shoulder muscles, she worked to release tight muscles around the capsule and, by pressing directly on the capsule, broke up some of the scar tissue that gummed up the works. Adhesive capsulitis is a stubborn condition; it took several months of treatment before Joan's frozen shoulder was completely "thawed" and she was back on the courts. On this second go-round, for every hour on the court, she spent an hour in the gym, stretching and strengthening her body to handle the demands of her sport.

Why the shoulder capsule should behave this way—the tissues begin to stick together and stick to the muscles that pass over them—is something of a medical mystery. Without treatment to speed healing, the capsule is likely to "freeze" for the better part of a year, then gradually "thaw" for several years as the pain subsides and most, but not all, of the lost range of motion returns. Frozen shoulder mostly affects women in their middle decades, which suggests that declining sex hormones play a role. Pushing an out-of-shape shoulder through a lot of overhead movement seems to be one way to set yourself up for the condition. A course of anti-inflammatory injections may be helpful.

The surgical solution is to cut the scar tissue in the capsule, then, with the patient under anesthesia, force the arm through its full range of motion. It works, but as long as the manual approach yields results, there's no reason to subject the patient to the risk of general anesthesia.

Joint/Orthopedic

Rotator-Cuff Tears (Full-Thickness Tears)

A recent patient of Dr. Kelly's was a fireman who, when asleep on a beach, had an off-roading truck run over his shoulder. Dr. Kelly repaired the huge tear in the tendon of the supraspinatus muscle, and the man went back to his activities.

There are no hard-and-fast rules about when to surgically repair the rotator cuff. Dr. Kelly was the lead author of a 1995 study that found that some people with serious cuff tears could still lift their arms over their head. Their strong muscles adequately compensated for the structural damage. Remember, just because something is broken doesn't necessarily mean it needs to be fixed!

For people in their eighties or nineties, it may be easier and wiser to adapt to physical limitations—don't put the cereal on the top shelf—than to deal with the rigors of surgery and rehab. For a guy in his thirties who installs Sheetrock for a living, a fully operational shoulder, or close to it, is his paycheck, and surgery is usually a given. The younger the patient and the better overall condition of the tendon, the better the odds for a successful surgery and a full recovery.

Shoulder Separation

As a lot of football and hockey players know firsthand, a sharp blow to the shoulder can sprain and even rupture the acromioclavicular (AC) ligament, which binds the collarbone (clavicle) to the broad tip of the shoulder blade (acromion process). In plain English, a shoulder separation. Most cases, with the help of RICE, heal on their own. The most serious ruptures may require surgical reconstruction of the AC joint to allow the arm to be lifted normally above the head, but surgery on this joint is not common.

Shoulder Dislocation

A recent college grad, Dan plays in a New Jersey recreational rugby league. His shoulder had never given him any problems until an opposing player slammed into his upper body when he was facedown on the field. He suffered a traumatic disloca-tion. Both Dan the rugby player and Laura the swimmer have unstable shoulders. But he needs surgery and she needs therapy to correct a muscle imbalance.

If your shoulder dislocates as the result of trauma, even partially (it's called a subluxation), it's time to see an orthopedist. The labrum, a ring of fibrocartilage that deepens the socket and helps keep the ball in place, often tears. The ball, or humeral head, can scrape against the socket, dislodging a wedge of cartilage. These are two good reasons younger people with normal shoulder anatomy who suffer a single traumatic dislocation have up to a 90 percent chance of suffering more dislocations if the damage isn't repaired. In many cases, labral tears in the shoulder require surgery. An unstable shoulder can lead to osteoarthritis down the road.

In some cases, as with partial tears of the rotator cuff, if you can decrease the symptoms by improving muscle function, you can avoid surgery even though a structural problem is still present. In the case of a labral tear, you may need sur-gery even if the pain goes away. Degenerative changes can occur over time if the shoulder is left untreated. Your orthopedist can help you to decide on a course of action.

Osteoarthritis

Shoulder arthritis isn't as common, or usually as debilitating, as arthritis in the knee or hip, but the shoulder is still vulnerable, at both the AC joint and the ball and socket joint. Because doctors don't yet know how to stop the overgrowth of the bone tissue, our options are limited. Manual therapy that relaxes the muscles and decreases the pressure of muscle tendons pulling on the joint can ease pain and stiffness and may prolong the life of a joint. Anti-inflammatory drugs and cortico-steroid injections, as long as they're not overprescribed, can be helpful. Severe cases of osteoarthritis can call for more aggressive measures if the patient is other-wise healthy enough to tolerate surgery. For the glenohumeral joint, that would be

Dr. Kelly

I have a patient, Rebecca, a forty-year-old woman who fell down and shattered the top part of her humerus, her upper-arm bone. A trauma surgeon came in and pieced the bone back together. So the bone fracture was fixed, but the shoulder joint and the muscles were a disaster. Her shoulder joint collapsed because the accident had cut off the blood supply to the area and the surrounding muscles had shut down. She was in excruciating pain and became addicted to narcotic pain meds. We removed the dead bone and converted her to a ball-and-socket shoulder prosthesis. She's got her life back.

joint replacement, replacing damaged bone and cartilage with a metal-and-plastic implant. For the AC joint, the procedure entails cutting away a portion of the collarbone and leaving a space between the bone and the tip of the shoulder blade. Some AC joint injuries may be repaired through surgical reconstruction.

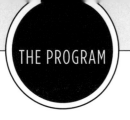

SHOULDER

The shoulder is arguably the most mobile joint in the body, but for this privilege it sacrifices stability. It is held together more by soft tissue than solid bony connection, so it is important that the tissue is maintained. All possible movements are achievable by the shoulder: flexion, extension, adduction, abduction, circumduction, and coupled movements (forward, back, toward you, out to the side, in a circle, and combinations of these). If you've ever seen a baseball pitch, a tennis swing, a gymnastic rings event, or a Cirque du Soleil performance, you can start to appreciate what the shoulder can do.

ANTERIOR UPPER ARM

Purpose: To target and remove any restrictions and restore a full range of motion to the three zones of the biceps by manually releasing tight, short, and damaged muscle fibers.

Starting out: Stand or sit with the feet spread shoulders' width apart. Raise the elbow and bring the hand toward the shoulder with a relaxed arm. Using the hand opposite the treatment side, place the thumb on the muscle with angled pressure. The three treatment zones are the inside, middle, and outside aspects of the biceps. Use the thumb for the inside zone and the fingertips to contact the middle and outside zones. If it is easier, use your fingers for all three zones.

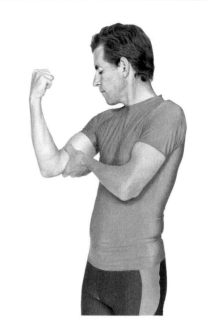

How to do it: Start by pressing on the muscle with either the thumb or the fingers (depending on your comfort and what zone you are treating). Then, use angled pressure as you straighten the treatment arm and bring it down next to the body. Keep the motion slow and controlled. Repeat with your other arm. Do two to three passes in each zone, starting each zone closer to the elbow and working toward the shoulder.

Troubleshooting: The muscle should be relaxed when the pressure is applied. Don't press too hard as this can irritate the muscle. Avoid letting the skin slide under the fingers by using constant, angled pressure.

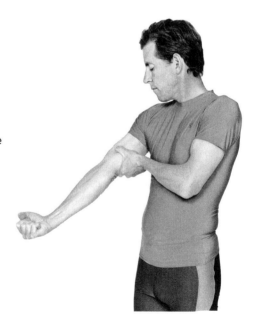

POSTERIOR UPPER ARM

Purpose: To target and remove any restrictions and restore a full range of motion to the three zones of the triceps by manually releasing tight, short, and damaged muscle fibers.

Starting out: Stand or sit with your feet spread shoulders' width apart. Straighten your arm down, with the palm facing up and the back of the arm relaxed. Using the opposite hand, place your thumb or fingertips on the muscle with angled pressure toward the shoulder. The three treatment zones are the inside, back, and outside aspects of the triceps. Use the fingertips with the palm up for the outside, or lateral zone, then flip the hand to use the thumb for the rest.

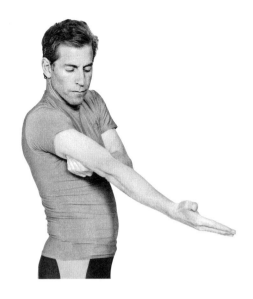

How to do it: Once contact is made, bend the elbow and raise the arm so that the elbow moves toward the ear. Keep the motion slow and controlled. Repeat with your other arm. Do two to three passes in each zone, starting each zone closer to the elbow and working toward the shoulder.

Troubleshooting: The muscle should be relaxed when the pressure is applied. Don't press too hard as this can irritate the muscle. Avoid letting the skin slide under the fingers by using constant, angled pressure. Maintain good posture—keep your head neutral.

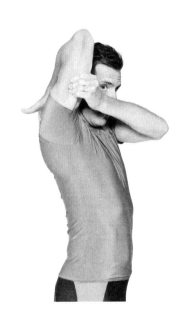

TOP OF THE SHOULDER

Purpose: To target and remove any restrictions and restore a full range of motion to the three zones of the supraspinatus.

Starting out: Sit on a stability ball with your feet spread shoulders' width apart. Straighten and raise your arm straight in front, with the palm facing up. The head is neutral and the face forward. Reach the opposite hand across the chest and place your fingertips on the muscle with angled pressure. The three treatment zones are the front, top or middle, and back aspects of the supraspinatus—a muscle between the neck and the shoulder. This muscle is deep to the upper trapezius.

How to do it: Angle the pressure in and toward the neck with your fingers. Once contact is made, bring the arm down, turn the palm around, and, reaching behind you, place the back of the hand over the opposite buttock. Tilt your head away from the treatment side, bringing the ear to the shoulder. Keep the motion slow and controlled. Repeat with your other arm. Do two to three passes in each zone, starting each zone closer to the neck and working toward the shoulder.

Troubleshooting: The muscle should be relaxed when the pressure is applied. Don't press too hard as this can irritate the muscle. Avoid letting the skin slide under the fingers by using constant, angled pressure. Move your arm through its full range of motion before engaging your hand. Don't shrug your shoulders.

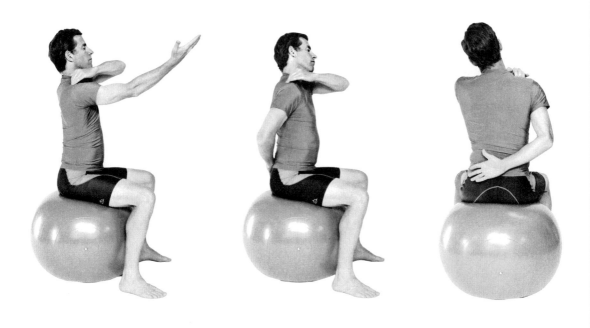

POSTERIOR SHOULDER

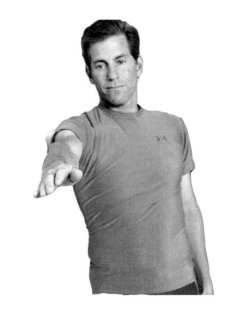

Purpose: To target and remove any restrictions and restore a full range of motion to the posterior deltoid and infraspinatus by manually releasing tight, short, and damaged muscles.

Starting out: Stand with your feet spread shoulders' width apart, and your body positioned at a forty-five-degree angle to a wall so that only the back of the shoulder touches it. Place a small, hard ball between your shoulder and the wall. The treatment-side arm should be extended straight out, parallel to the wall. Lean slightly into the ball so that it presses comfortably into the back of your shoulder.

How to do it: Maintaining pressure with a slight lean, move the treatment arm across the body, not letting it or the ball drop. Use the opposite arm to gently bring the treatment arm through its range of motion. Hold for a count of two. Repeat with your other arm. Do two to three repetitions, releasing and moving the ball to a slightly different place each time.

Troubleshooting: Don't press too hard as this can irritate the muscle. Avoid letting the skin slide under the ball—this might be a little harder than with your hand or fingers. There is a learning curve with this move. Be patient as it may take several attempts to perfect it.

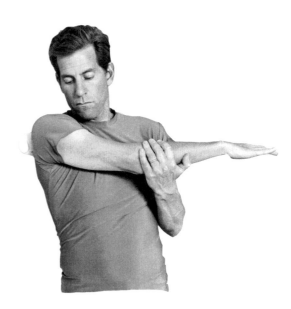

ANTERIOR SHOULDER

Purpose: To target and remove any restrictions and restore a full range of motion to the pectoral muscles and the anterior deltoid by manually releasing tight, short, and damaged muscles.

Starting out: Sit or stand with your feet spread shoulders' width apart. The treatment arm should be neutral and relaxed (you can even rest it in your lap). With the other hand, apply angled pressure down and in at the area where the shoulder and chest come together (your pressure should pull slightly down and across the body).

How to do it: Maintaining pressure across the body, straighten the treatment arm back and away from the shoulder. Bring the fingers back to open the palm, and tilt your face away from the treatment area. Hold for a count of two. Repeat with your other arm. Do two to three repetitions, releasing and moving the hand from point to point along the one treatment zone from the shoulder to the chest.

Troubleshooting: Don't press too hard as this can irritate the muscles. Avoid letting the skin slide under the fingers by using constant, angled pressure. Be gentle with the thin muscle over the shoulder joint itself.

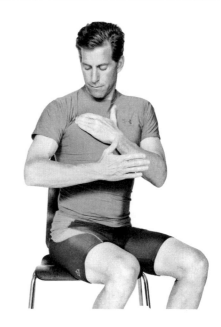

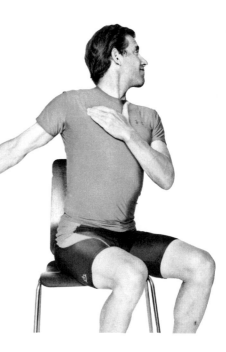

UPPER POSTERIOR ARM

Purpose: To bring the posterior upper-arm muscles (the triceps especially, but also the latissimi dorsi, the teres muscles, the lower traps, and the pectoralis muscles) through their pain-free range of motion. This will warm them up and allow the ends of the ROM to be safely explored.

Starting out: Stand with your feet spread shoulders' width apart and your elbow bent. Cup the elbow with the opposite hand.

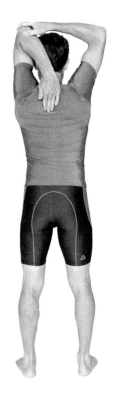

How to do it: Bring the elbow up, guided gently by the other hand, and slide the treatment hand (palm side in) down the back as far as is comfortable. Keep the opposite arm lifted so that it frames the head by the end of the movement. This should gently stretch the back of the arm and possibly the side of the body. Hold for a count of two. Repeat with your other arm. Do ten repetitions, held for no more than two seconds each.

Troubleshooting: Don't overdo this stretch. Stop before you feel any uncomfortable compression in the shoulder joint. Keep both shoulders down and a good, relaxed posture.

POSTERIOR SHOULDER MUSCLES

Purpose: To bring the posterior shoulder muscles (posterior deltoid, infraspinatus, rhomboids, latissimi dorsi, and the middle and lower trapezius) through their pain-free range of motion.

Starting out: Sit or stand with your feet spread shoulders' width apart and your arm extended to the side. Maintain an upright posture, with the shoulder, elbow, and hand all in one line parallel to the floor.

How to do it: Bring your arm across the body, using the opposite hand to gently bring the elbow toward the opposite shoulder. You should feel a stretch in the back of the shoulder and into the back. Hold for a count of two. Repeat with your other arm. Do ten repetitions, held for no more than two seconds each.

Troubleshooting: Don't crunch the shoulder when pulling with the opposite hand. Keep both shoulders down and a good, relaxed posture.

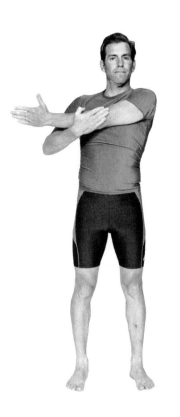

ANTERIOR SHOULDER MUSCLES

Purpose: To bring the anterior shoulder muscles (anterior deltoid, pectoralis major and minor, and subscapularis) through their pain-free range of motion. This will warm them up and allow the ends of the ROM to be safely explored. This is a great stretch for everybody.

Starting out: Stand with your feet spread shoulders' width apart, your shoulder and elbow in a line parallel to the floor, and your hand raised so that it's directly above the elbow. The elbow and hand should both be lined up on the inside of a doorway.

How to do it: Keeping the arm still, turn the head and body away from the arm. There should be a gentle stretch in the front of the shoulder and into the chest. Hold for a count of two. Repeat with your other arm. Do ten repetitions, held for no more than two seconds each.

Troubleshooting: Don't let your elbow drop. Keep both shoulders down in a relaxed posture. Don't overtwist the body, only go to a comfortable position. Discontinue if you feel pain.

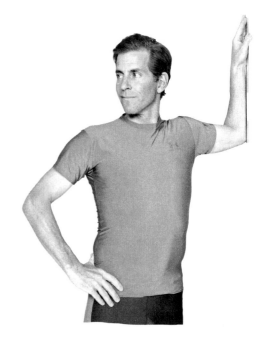

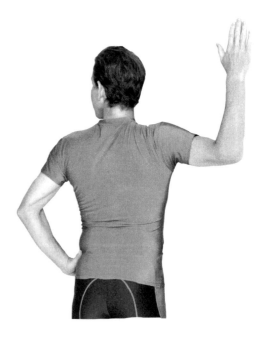

TOP OF THE SHOULDER AND POSTERIOR SHOULDER

Purpose: To strengthen the muscles of external shoulder rotation. This includes a complex movement pattern of muscles: the supra- and infraspinatus, the three trapezius muscles, the posterior and middle deltoids, the rhomboids, and a host of stabilizers. This will warm them up and increase shoulder stabilization.

Starting out: Stand with your feet shoulders' width apart. The treatment arm should be straight and across the body, with the hand gripping a flex-band or weight at the opposite hip. The tension of the flex-band should be coming from the floor at the side opposite to the treatment side.

How to do it: Holding the flex-band or weight, and keeping the arm straight, bring the arm out, up, and across the body, so that the hand ends up in line with, or slightly above, the head. Squeeze the shoulder blades in and down to help achieve this. Repeat with your other arm. Do ten repetitions, held for no more than two seconds each.

Troubleshooting: Do not let the shoulders ride up or keep your neck tense. Keep the arm straight throughout the movement. Remember to squeeze your shoulders blades back and down at the end of each repetition, and keep your back engaged and upright. Don't use stretch cords or weights that are too resistant or heavy.

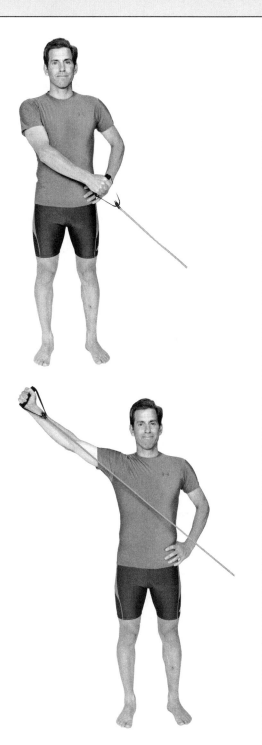

POSTERIOR SHOULDER

Purpose: To strengthen and return function to the muscles of external shoulder rotation: infraspinatus, posterior deltoid, and teres minor. There are fewer dedicated external rotators, so it is important to keep them in balance with the internal rotators. This will warm them up and increase shoulder stabilization. This is an important exercise for posture, and to counteract the effects of computer work, driving—any activity where the arms work in front of the body.

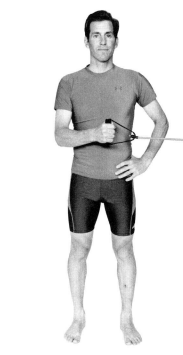

Starting out: Stand with your feet shoulders' width apart. The treatment arm should be bent with the elbow touching your side and the forearm parallel to the floor. The elbow and shoulder should be pivoted toward the opposite side as far as is possible without losing the contact between the elbow and the body. The grip of a flex-band should be held in the hand, with the tension of the flex-band coming from the opposite side at the same height as the hand.

How to do it: Pivot the arm at the shoulder and elbow toward the treatment side of your body, keeping the hand parallel to the floor and the elbow touching your side. Squeeze the shoulder blades in and down to help achieve this. Repeat with your other arm. Do ten repetitions, held for no more than two seconds each. If no flex-band is available, the same exercise can be done with a hand weight in a side-lying position.

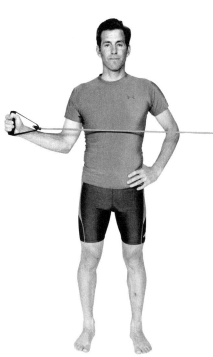

Troubleshooting: Do not let your shoulders ride up or tense your neck. Remember to squeeze the shoulders back at the end of each repetition. Don't use the rest of your body by twisting or leaning.

ANTERIOR SHOULDER

Purpose: To strengthen the muscles of internal shoulder rotation and to return proper function to the anterior deltoid, subscapularis, coracobrachialis, and pectoralis major, and to improve their interaction. This will warm them up and increase shoulder stabilization.

Starting out: Stand with your feet shoulders' width apart. The treatment arm should be bent with the elbow touching your side and the forearm parallel to the floor. Squeeze the shoulder blades in and down to help achieve this. The grip of a flex-band should be held in your hand, with the tension of the flex-band coming from the treatment side at the same height as the hand.

How to do it: Pivot the arm at the shoulder and move the hand toward the opposite side of the body, keeping the hand parallel to the floor and the elbow touching your side. Repeat with your other arm. Do ten repetitions, held for no more than two seconds each. If no flex-band is available, the same exercise can be done with a hand weight in a side-lying position.

Troubleshooting: Do not let the shoulders ride up or tense the neck. Remember to squeeze the shoulders back at the start of each repetition. Don't use the rest of your body by twisting or leaning.

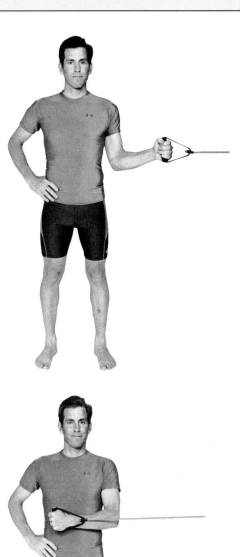

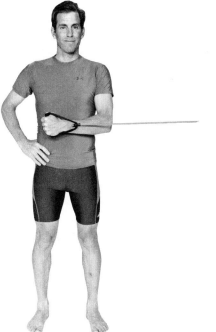

THE ELBOW/WRIST/HAND

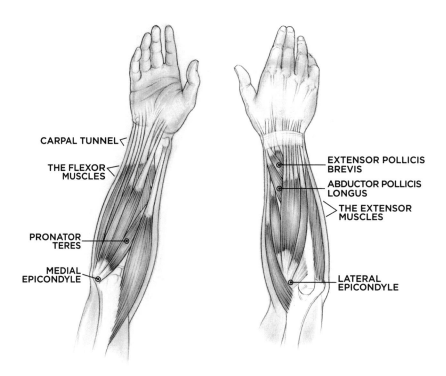

CARPAL TUNNEL

THE FLEXOR
MUSCLES

PRONATOR
TERES

MEDIAL
EPICONDYLE

EXTENSOR POLLICIS
BREVIS

ABDUCTOR POLLICIS
LONGUS

THE EXTENSOR
MUSCLES

LATERAL
EPICONDYLE

INTRODUCING THE ELBOW/WRIST/HAND

Outside of the brain itself, the elbow, wrist, and hand, with its opposable thumb, comprise the area of the body that best defines us as human. The flexibility of our upper extremities, culminating in those dexterous hands, have helped drive the evolution of our problem-solving species . . . and given us the modern tools that we sometimes overuse and misuse to wind up in pain.

When we talk about issues at the elbow, wrist, and hand we're mostly talking about overuse injuries. Typically when you wield a computer mouse or a screwdriver or a tennis racquet for hours on end, you forget to use the leverage of the whole upper body. The muscles of the neck and shoulder grow fatigued and tense from *not* moving, and the smaller muscles in the forearms tire from performing repeated small movements without a break. Clicking on a computer mouse seems so innocuous that you don't realize you've overdone it until the muscles have been pushed over the edge into irritation and inflammation. Then you can't bend your wrist or elbow without wincing. These overuse injuries, sometimes labeled repetitive stress injuries or RSIs, are the bane of both the work and sports worlds. Lateral epicondylitis (tennis elbow) is one of the most common upper-extremity musculoskeletal complaints and carpal tunnel syndrome the most notorious workplace injury, both contributing to the many millions that RSIs cost the nation in medical care, lost wages, worker's compensation, and other indirect expenses.

RED FLAG

IMMEDIATE TREATMENT/ WHEN TO SEE A DOCTOR

Chronic injury that includes shooting pain and numbness usually means nerve involvement and should be looked at by a doctor. Prolonged numbness and muscle weakening are signs of a serious problem. Trauma to the wrist that results in pain and swelling should be checked out by a doctor. Older people often suffer severe sprains and fractures after a fall; these injuries require splinting or casting to heal properly. As with any joint problem, check for any signs of infection—redness, heat or fever, pain not connected to changes in activity. If there are any, see a doctor immediately. When the dire possibilities have been ruled out, you can assume you have some less serious form of soft-tissue damage such as a mild ligament sprain or a muscle/tendon strain. The normal rules of RICE apply: Rest (keep weight off the area); Ice it; keep inflammation down with Compression (a compression bandage); and Elevation (bring the affected area above the level of your heart).

In the forearm, as in the spine, a lot is going on in a relatively cramped space: muscles, tendons, and nerves are moving together in close proximity. That's a recipe for nerves getting compressed, triggering pain and dysfunction. Once again, it pays to analyze what goes wrong in terms of the three major elements of the system: bones, joints, and muscles. Let's take the popular diagnosis of carpal tunnel syndrome (CTS): it's a set of symptoms created when the median nerve is compressed within the carpal tunnel. This sounds plausible and it gets a lot of attention in the media, so people with numb, achy hands are often convinced they have it. We agree with our colleague at the Hospital for Special Surgery, physiatrist Dr. Jennifer Solomon (see the box on page 89), that CTS is overdiagnosed. Many, perhaps most, cases are caused by tight muscles clamping down on the nerve above the wrist. In these cases, manual therapy to relax the muscles works wonders; surgery to release pressure on the median nerve (the standard remedy for severe CTS cases) needn't be considered.

If we are to achieve complex movement patterns, the movement of individual body parts must be coordinated. The resulting sequence of movement is called a kinetic chain. Trouble high on the chain usually translates to trouble below. The arm is a perfect example. The shoulder muscles act on the shoulder joint to move the upper arm, the upper-arm muscles act on the elbow to move the forearm, the forearm acts on the wrist to move the hand. The elbow joint, the middle link in the chain, is pretty straightforward. The single bone of the upper arm, the humerus, meets the two bones of the forearm, the radius and ulna, at the elbow. The longer ulna fits into the humerus to create a one-way hinge: it opens, it closes. The shorter radius pivots on the ulna and humerus next to that hinge, allowing you to twist your forearm. The elbow is held together by ligaments and protected by the bony protuberance of the humerus.

The wrist is more complicated. At the opposite end from the elbow, the radius and the ulna come together to cradle a row of four irregularly shaped wrist bones. In front of them lies another row of four bones, all together, the carpals. The whole system is tied together by a series of small, flexible ligaments that give the hand/wrist unit its unparalleled versatility. The wrist flexes forward and back and from side to side. Just beneath the underside of the wrist is the transverse carpal ligament, which forms one wall of the famously crowded carpal tunnel of bones and connective tissue through which passes veins, arteries, three major nerves, and the tendons of the four fingers and the thumb muscles.

COMMON PROBLEMS AND CULPRITS

The muscles that power the forearm—the biceps and brachialis in the front of the arm that flex the elbow, and the triceps in the back that straighten it out—are big guns that don't overload easily. But people do strain or tear the biceps by lifting heavy objects. Weight-room regulars can overdevelop the biceps at the expense of the triceps, setting themselves up for imbalance injuries.

The smaller muscles of the forearm that control the wrist and hand are the most likely candidates for repetitive stress injuries. The extensor muscles that run down the back of the forearm pull the wrist back, or "extend" it, as the name implies. Repetitive motion at work (wielding a screwdriver or a scalpel, for instance) or at play (tennis, bowling) can irritate and inflame the muscles and tendons, creating what we call lateral epicondylitis or "tennis elbow." Repeatedly flexing the wrist does the same number on the flexor muscles that run along the front of the arm and attach at the inside knob of the elbow, the medial epicondyle. Golfers, bowlers, baseball pitchers, and people who work with their hands can suffer the somewhat less common "golfer's elbow," or medial epicondylitis.

Two forearm muscles that control the thumb, the abductor pollicis longus and extensor pollicis brevis, can fatigue and shorten, irritating and inflaming their common tendon and tendon sheath, causing pain on the thumb side of the wrist. This overuse condition, De Quervain's syndrome, often afflicts people who take up potentially thumb-stressing activities such as knitting or prolonged computer use, or new mothers who are constantly picking up their infants.

The most frequently diagnosed nerve disorder in the arm is carpal tunnel syndrome. The median nerve passes through the carpal tunnel, where it can be compressed. This compression can cause numbness, tingling, and weakness in the thumb, index, or middle fingers, as well as the palm and forearm. Space in the tunnel gets tight when, for example, repetitive stress causes the neighboring tendons to become inflamed or the transverse carpal ligament thickens. But tight muscles, typically the pronator teres, which helps rotate the forearm, often compress the nerve and create the exact same symptoms. The ulnar nerve, which passes through a groove on the inside of the elbow (at the medial epicondyle), can also become compressed, causing tingling and numbness in the fourth and fifth fingers—a sister syndrome to CTS known as cubital tunnel syndrome. Like the median nerve, the ulnar nerve can be compressed by tight muscles at a number of spots up and down the arm. The radial nerve can suffer the same fate, getting trapped at several sites in the arm, causing numbness and tingling on the back of the hand.

WHAT GOES WRONG, AND HOW TO FIX IT

Mostly Muscular

Tennis Elbow (Lateral Epicondylitis)

Bob is a fifty-seven-year-old teaching tennis pro in northern New Jersey who has been treated for tennis elbow off and on for over a decade. He's received corticosteroid injections for the trouble spot, which helped for a little while, until the next flare-up, when the outer side of the elbow would again become painfully tender. Bob has a classic overuse injury. The forearm muscles that constantly work to straighten out the elbow (for instance, hitting backhand shots over and over) get irritated, along with the tendon on the outside of the elbow to which they are attached. The muscle medicine approach is to manually work to relax the muscles of the forearm that are tugging on that tendon and, in Bob's case, to work on the tight shoulder that was contributing to the problem. He was out of trouble after six visits. Then he was able to begin physical therapy to strengthen the muscles that supported his newfound normal range of motion in the shoulder. He's been pain-free for the past two years.

We actually don't like the label *tennis elbow*. Therapists and physicians see lots of lateral epicondylitis patients who play tennis and lots who don't. What they all tend to have in common is poor form doing their chosen activity. Often the problem begins at the shoulder—think of it as the first domino to fall. If the shoulder muscles are tight and the shoulder joint is not able to rotate normally, the elbow and wrist will have to make up the difference with extra motion, in this case over-extension. That's true whether you're hitting a backhand or taking care of home repairs with a screwdriver. Muscle imbalance can be another contributing factor. If the biceps is tight or overdeveloped, the antagonist muscle, the triceps will have to overwork to straighten out the elbow, stressing that same outer-elbow area.

Golfer's elbow, or medial epicondylitis, is a similar story, except this time it's the flexor muscles and tendons on the front of the forearm that attach to the inner knob of the elbow, the medial epicondyle, that get overstressed. Golfers, bowlers, and baseball pitchers, who flex or snap their wrists, are vulnerable, as are people who put in long hours working with hand tools.

The textbook explanation of what happens in these tendinitis cases is that overstressed tendons and muscles suffer repeated microscopic tears that lead to inflammation. It's inflammation that the *itis* in *lateral epicondylitis* or *Achilles tendinitis* refers to. As we mentioned in chapter 3, researchers now understand that tendons, unlike muscles, have only a limited capacity to become inflamed. With chronic tendinitis, the initial swelling goes away. It is more likely that the pain is caused by the repeated scarring of the tendon or irritating chemicals produced by that scarring. Both of these reduce the blood supply and make the tissue brittle and more susceptible to further injury. (*Tendonosis* is a better term for this degeneration of the tendon's collagen fibers, but the medical profession has been slow to update its vocabulary.) Manual therapy works because it reduces the muscle's pull on the tendon, allowing the tendon some relief from tension so it can heal. Meanwhile, leading doctors in academic medicine have been rethinking the medical treatment of damaged tendons (see the box below). For those uncommon cases of tennis elbow and golfer's elbow that resist all forms of conservative treatment, surgical procedures can remove the damaged section of the tendon and stitch it back together.

INFO

PRP THERAPY

Dr. Jennifer Solomon, physiatrist, Hospital for Special Surgery: "Lots of doctors try to treat chronic tendon pain with corticosteroid injections to reduce inflammation, but patients may not necessarily respond. Most of the pain associated with tendonosis probably comes not from inflammation but from other irritating biochemical substances associated with the injury. It's more important to address the underlying issue. For a majority of cases, doing manual muscle therapy and then physical therapy is highly effective. But there are patients for whom nothing seems to work. With this group, we are having a lot of success with PRP or plasma-enriched protein injections. We take some of the person's blood, thin it down to obtain nutrient-rich plasma, and inject it back into the area. It gets nutrients into the tendon tissue and promotes healing. I think in the next ten years you're going to see it being used to treat arthritis, spinal disks, a lot of musculoskeletal areas where we hadn't had much progress before."

De Quervain's Tenosynovitis

Ruth, in her fifties, worked at an assembly-line job in a New Jersey factory, where she performed the same movement over and over, hooking a metal plate with a device and flipping it over. After years of that, she had developed a persistent dull ache on the thumb side of her wrist. This was De Quervain's tenosynovitis, an inflammation and irritation of the tendon sheath that houses several small muscles that control the thumb. Her doctor put her in a wrist brace, which offered no relief. He gave her a corticosteroid injection, which did relieve her symptoms, but only for a few months, because the tight, shortened muscles weren't addressed. Finally, manual therapy broke up the tightness in the muscles that were pulling on the tendon, and this relieved the pain. Once the muscles could move normally, Ruth was given conditioning exercises to develop the strength and flexibility of the muscles and tendons. On her own time, she was able to build up the resilience of the forearm so she could return to her job without crossing the line into repetitive stress injury.

Painstaking manual work such as sewing or woodworking or, in Ruth's case, assembly-line labor requires twisting and grasping movements that can overstress the thumb tendons, especially when the wrist is held in an extended position (knuckle side pulled back).

With any new activity, the muscles and tendons may not have a chance to adjust to the sudden extra demand. Baby-holding isn't exactly a sport, but good form is just as important as it is in tennis. When De Quervain's is caught early enough, inflammation is part of the injury package; Dr. Solomon has had good success treating it with one or two corticosteroid injections. But the best plan of attack is the same as with the other repetitive stress arm injuries: correct your form, relax the muscles manually, and condition them with physical therapy exercises.

Muscle or Joint?

Carpal Tunnel Syndrome

Julie is a twenty-five-year-old grad student at Rutgers, anxiously typing through the day, trying to finish her dissertation on deadline. As she neared her goal, her hands began to give out on her. She's had numbness and tingling in the thumb and first two fingers of her left hand. A diagnostic test revealed she had a mild case of carpal tunnel syndrome. Her doctor recommended surgery, but she was willing to try the

PROTECT YOUR WRISTS

When you're typing, you should be able to keep your wrists straight and your elbows bent at about ninety degrees. A sliding keyboard tray can help you find the right distance between the keyboard and your body. Try to keep your forearms in a neutral position and not slightly turned out to either side.

When you're typing or doing housework or home repairs that involve a lot of wrist movement, take breaks as often as possible, for instance, every fifteen minutes or half an hour.

Whether you're picking up a baby or working a screwdriver, keep your arms in as close to the body as you can. The more you extend the arms, the more stress you're putting on the elbow and wrist.

If you have any hand/wrist nerve issues, try wearing a wrist splint or brace to bed. People often sleep in a stressful, wrist-flexed position.

Tennis players and golfers should get regular tune-ups from a teaching pro, especially if they're having elbow or wrist pain. Tennis players with tennis elbow should take a look at their racquet. A racquet that is too heavy, too tightly strung, or has too small a grip may be causing or contributing to the problem.

Don't lean on your elbows.

Weight lifters who pump up their biceps need to make sure to develop balance by working the antagonist muscle, the triceps, as well.

muscle medicine approach first. Dr. DeStefano worked to loosen all the muscles in the shoulder and the forearm, but as he suspected, it was a small forearm muscle, the pronator teres, that was the primary problem. The tight, inflamed muscle had been pressing against the median nerve. After five visits, Dr. DeStefano had restored normal movement to the muscle and the symptoms disappeared. Julie went home with a program of stretching and strengthening exercises to keep her out of trouble as she plowed through the last chapters of her dissertation.

In her fifties, Martha had kept up a heavy daily typing schedule for two decades working as a secretary for a northern New Jersey manufacturing company. She'd had intermittent pain and numbness in the hands for years, but she'd managed to get by, dulling the symptoms with Advil. Finally, it became too much. She was

manually treated for the muscles of her arm, wrist, and hand, including the prona-
tor teres, but she improved only slightly. The nerve damage was so severe that the
muscles in the hand that are activated by the median nerve had already started to
weaken, or atrophy. She couldn't open a jar and could barely button her shirt. Dr.
DeStefano sent her to a hand specialist who cut the transverse carpal ligament and
opened up badly needed space for the nerve. The operation was a success, but she
still had some localized hand pain caused by surgical scarring. Manual work on the
scarred muscle tissue brought her completely out of pain.

Two stories, two different strategies. Overuse injuries often come about from a combination of different factors. In the case of carpal tunnel syndrome, the main issue is the pressure on the median nerve within the carpal tunnel. But the median nerve can be entrapped by the transverse carpal ligament directly, by the swelling of structures within the tunnel, or by an accumulation of scar tissue or foreign bodies.

Again, it comes down to that combination of bone, joint, and muscle that is specific to every person's injury. Both Julie and Martha were women with narrow wrist bones, which made them even more susceptible. (Pregnancy, and the fluid retention that comes with it, is another risk factor; genetics and trauma, which don't discriminate by gender, can also bring the syndrome on.) Julie is young. Her con-

INFO

DR. JENNIFER SOLOMON ON CARPAL TUNNEL SYNDROME

Carpal tunnel syndrome is overdiagnosed. I have patients coming in—a lot of secretaries—and they have numbness and tingling in the fingers. They're convinced they need carpal tunnel surgery. I do a nerve conduction study that measures how fast the nerve signal travels down the median nerve, and the results are normal. I send them to Rob and he works to release the pronator teres muscle, and their symptoms dramatically improve. Of course, sometimes the transverse carpal tunnel really is compressing the nerve, or there is a problem within the tunnel. Then they are surgical candidates. But surgery always has risks—scarring, infection, nerve or muscle damage. Some hand specialists do really well with these patients using wrists splints and a corticosteroid injection.

nective tissue is in its supple prime, and she had a relatively short history of repetitive stress. So it wasn't surprising that the joint structure was only mildly damaged. We could solve her problem by addressing the tight muscles that were irritating the tendons and the muscle compressing the median nerve. (The muscle had become overstressed by Julie's tendency to twist her left arm inward when she typed.) Martha, on the other hand, had everything working against her. When the connection between nerve and muscle is that frayed, surgery is the usual solution. Without it, nerve fibers can die, leaving muscles permanently disabled.

Other patients require a different selection of "tools" from the "toolbox." Often, bad work habits and bad keyboard/mouse ergonomics need to be corrected (see the Self-Defense box on page 131). Wrist splints and braces used to be a popular way to try to take pressure off the carpal tunnel area. We, and most experts in the field, now agree that immobilizing the arm muscles at work all day is a bad idea. However, wearing splints to bed can work well for patients whose wrists naturally assume a stressful, flexed position.

Ulnar Nerve Entrapment/Cubital Tunnel Syndrome

Everyone has had the experience of banging their funny bone on the inside of the elbow. Not very funny at all. The ulnar nerve, which passes by the elbow close to the surface of the skin, triggers all that pain and tingling. The ulnar nerve is one of three major nerves that pass down the arm and through the wrist. Like the median nerve getting trapped in the carpal tunnel, the ulnar nerve can get compressed in a tunnel in the hand called the tunnel of Guyon. But it's more likely to run into problems at the elbow by getting squeezed into a groove in the funny bone (ulna) known as the cubital tunnel, which can cause tingling and numbness in the fourth and little fingers. A very successful surgical procedure can reposition the ulnar nerve away from the cubital tunnel, but manual therapy to release tight muscles up and down the arm can often help resolve the problem. Often, a bottleneck at the joint is not the crux of the problem. The ulnar nerve can be compressed by tight muscles at a number of spots on the arm, but a commonly overlooked area is in the shoulder region at the subscapularis, where the nerve originates (as the medial cord of the brachial plexus).

Joint/Orthopedic

Sprained Wrist

A sprained wrist is the most common wrist injury and is often serious. We see it in elderly patients who try to break a fall with their outstretched arms and in athletes, who usually have some help being driven to the ground. Ligaments on either side of the wrist can sprain, and the area becomes tender and painful. A wrist splint or plaster cast may be necessary, and a severe ligament tear may require surgery.

Wrist Fracture

Without an X-ray, it's often difficult to tell whether you've sprained a ligament or suffered a fracture of the ulna or radius bone in the forearm or the scaphoid bone of the wrist. The scaphoid fracture is more common and more serious. It may require a splint or a cast, and because the scaphoid-bone area has such a poor blood supply, surgical repair is a possible worst-case scenario. Women and seniors of both sexes should get a bone-density test if they've been diagnosed with a wrist fracture. Bone thinning, or osteoporosis, could be the underlying problem.

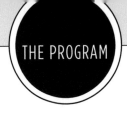

ELBOW/WRIST/ HAND

The motions at the wrist are flexion, extension, adduction, and abduction (bend forward, bend back, bend to the pinkie side, and bend to the thumb side), as well as circumduction. The movements at the elbow are simple flexion and extension.

ANTERIOR (PALM SIDE) OF THE FOREARM

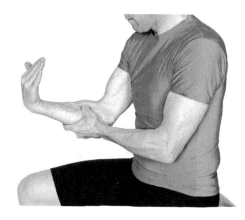

Purpose: To target and remove any restrictions and restore a full range of motion to the three zones of the flexor group by manually releasing tight, short, and damaged muscles. This is a great treatment for anyone who does repetitive movements with their hands or arms: from tennis to carpentry to computing.

Starting out: Sit on a stability ball or chair with your feet spread shoulders' width apart. Your palm should be facing up and flexed so that the fingers point toward the ceiling. Use the hand opposite to the treatment side and place the thumb, fingertips, or a ball or stick on the muscle, with pressure angled in and up toward the elbow. The three treatment zones are the inside, middle, and outside aspects of the flexor group. Use whatever hand position works best for you.

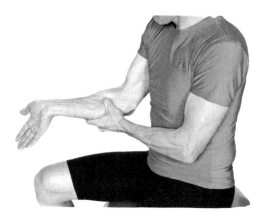

How to do it: Once contact is made, bring the back of the hand toward the floor until the fingers are angled toward the floor, then straighten the elbow. Keep the motion slow and controlled. Repeat with your other arm. Do two to three passes in each zone, starting each zone closer to the wrist and working toward the elbow. To generate more pressure, you can use a golf or tennis ball.

Troubleshooting: The muscle should be relaxed when the pressure is applied. Don't press too hard as it can irritate the muscles. Avoid letting the skin slide under the fingers by using constant, angled pressure. Be sure to extend both the wrist and elbow for a complete stretch—some of these muscles cross both joints.

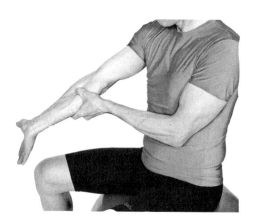

POSTERIOR (KNUCKLE SIDE) OF THE FOREARM

Purpose: To target and remove any restrictions and restore a full range of motion to the three zones of the extensor group by manually releasing tight, short, and damaged muscles.

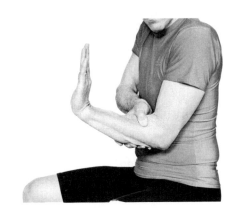

Starting out: Sit on a stability ball or chair with your feet spread shoulders' width apart. The back of your hand should be facing up and extended so that the fingers point toward the ceiling. Use the hand opposite to the treatment side and place the thumb, fingers, or edge of the hand (the karate-chop side) on the muscle. Apply angled pressure toward the elbow. The three treatment zones are the top, middle, and bottom aspects of the extensor group. Use whatever treatment position works best for you.

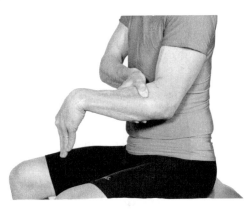

How to do it: Once contact is made, bring the palm of the treatment hand toward the floor, until the fingers are angled toward the floor. Keep the motion slow and controlled. Then extend the elbow so that the arm is straight. Repeat with your other arm. Do two to three passes in each zone, starting each zone closer to the elbow and working toward the wrist.

Troubleshooting: The muscles should be relaxed when the pressure is first applied. Don't press too hard as this can irritate the muscles. Avoid letting the skin slide under the fingers by using constant, angled pressure. Be sure to extend both the wrist and elbow for a complete stretch—some of the muscles cross both joints. When extending the elbow, it may be easier to use the fingers of the treatment hand instead of the thumb.

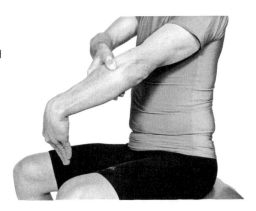

ANTERIOR (PALM SIDE) OF THE FOREARM

Purpose: To bring the flexor group through its pain-free range of motion. This will warm up the muscles and help relieve tension.

Starting out: Sit on a stability ball or chair with your feet spread shoulders' width apart. The treatment arm should be bent at the elbow with the hand palm up and in a neutral position. Your opposite hand should be holding the treatment hand with the fingers across the treatment fingers.

How to do it: Straighten your arm, then use the opposite hand to gently bring the fingers of the treatment hand back toward the body. Keep the motion slow and controlled. Hold for a count of two. Repeat with your other arm. Do ten repetitions, held for no more than two seconds each.

Troubleshooting: Don't pull on the muscles of the hand—you should feel no more than a gentle stretch. Less is more! Make sure the elbow is straight before extending the fingers.

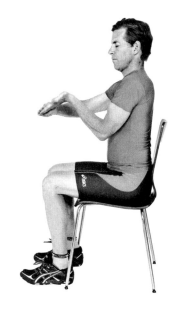

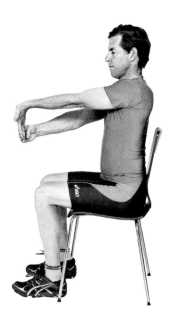

POSTERIOR (KNUCKLE SIDE) OF THE FOREARM

Purpose: To stretch the extensor group. This will help increase flexibility and prevent injury and tightness.

Starting out: While standing with your arm straight at your side, flex your wrist, stretching the muscles on the posterior side of the wrist.

How to do it: With the wrist still flexed, turn your fingers away from your body to feel the stretch in the extensor muscles of the forearm. Repeat with your other wrist.

Troubleshoot: Make sure to keep your wrist flexed and your elbow straight and locked throughout the stretch.

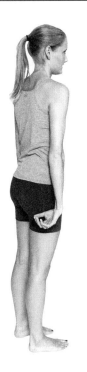

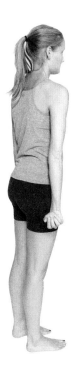

ANTERIOR (PALM SIDE) OF THE FOREARM

Purpose: Wrist curls, to strengthen the flexor group. This will warm up the muscles and help prevent strain on the structures of the wrist and forearm.

Starting out: Sit on a stability ball or chair with your feet spread shoulders' width apart. The treatment elbow should rest on the knee, with the palm facing up and the wrist extended. A hand weight should be held loosely.

How to do it: Grip the weight and curl it up toward your body, without taking the forearm off the leg. This isolates the target muscles. Hold for a count of two. Repeat with your other arm. Do ten repetitions, held for no more than two seconds each.

Troubleshooting: Make sure the rest of your body stays relaxed—keep the movement restricted to the forearm. Don't let the shoulders ride up and don't lift the forearm off the leg.

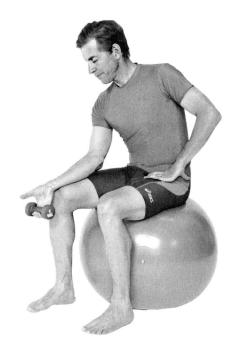

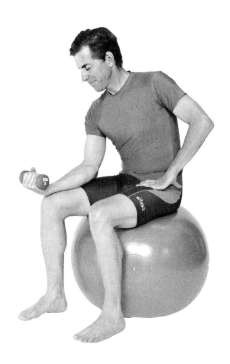

POSTERIOR (KNUCKLE SIDE) OF THE FOREARM

Purpose: Wrist extension, to strengthen the extensor group. This will warm up the muscles and help prevent strain on the structures of the forearm.

Starting out: Sit on a stability ball or chair with your feet spread shoulders' width apart. The treatment elbow should rest on the leg, with the palm facing down and the wrist flexed. A hand weight should be held loosely.

How to do it: Grip the weight and bring it up and toward the body by pulling the wrist back. Keep your forearm on the leg throughout the movement. Hold for a count of two. Repeat with your other arm. Do ten repetitions, held for no more than two seconds each.

Troubleshooting: Make sure the rest of your body stays relaxed—keep the movement restricted to the forearm. Don't let the shoulders ride up and don't lift the forearm off the leg.

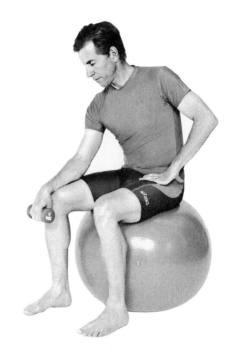

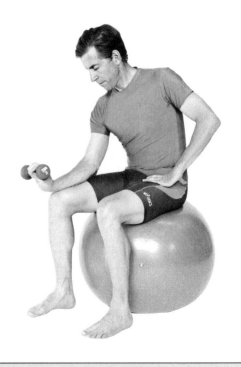

THE LOWER BACK

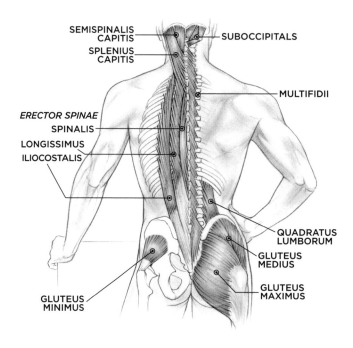

SEMISPINALIS CAPITIS

SUBOCCIPITALS

SPLENIUS CAPITIS

MULTIFIDII

ERECTOR SPINAE

SPINALIS

LONGISSIMUS

ILIOCOSTALIS

QUADRATUS LUMBORUM

GLUTEUS MEDIUS

GLUTEUS MAXIMUS

GLUTEUS MINIMUS

INTRODUCING THE LOWER BACK

No body "hot spot" is hotter than the lower back. Take a look at the statistics. At any given moment, as much as 20 percent of the human race is thought to be suffering from lower-back pain. Over their lifetime, the vast majority of Americans will experience at least one episode of back pain. Interestingly enough, in a majority of lower-back-pain cases, doctors are often unsure of the cause.

The lower back has its reasons for being so much trouble, juggling three demanding and sometimes conflicting jobs. The five vertebrae that make up the lumbar spine have to keep you upright while supporting most of your body weight. They have to provide some flexibility to the torso, otherwise you couldn't twist to the side or bend at the waist to tie your shoes. And they must provide safe housing for the spinal cord and the millions of nerve fibers that link every part of the body with the command center in the brain. As we discussed in chapter 8, aging makes this juggling act progressively more difficult.

For most people, from the twentysomethings on up, the area of greatest vulnerability in the lower-back hardware are the disks. The disks are the "jelly doughnuts" that fit in between the vertebrae—thick fibrocartilage on the outside, gel on the inside—that act as flexible shock absorbers throughout the length of the spine. (In the knee, the protective fibrocartilage is inside the joint, the meniscus.) After age forty, the interior gel begins to dehydrate and shrink, and the exterior disk is prone to cracking, or "herniating," which can irritate the surrounding nerves, muscles, or both.

Life dishes out plenty of abuse to the disks (see the boxes on pages 146 and 147 on protecting your lower back). After age forty or fifty, not too many people have a lumbar-spine MRI that's suitable for framing. But medical science still doesn't have a textbook explanation for the lower-back pain of patients who don't have glaring joint problems, or why the same amount of visible damage causes no problems in three people but the fourth person is in agony. By now, it won't surprise you to learn that we think the key to much lower-back pain is in the muscles.

The ligaments that run up and down the lumbar (and cervical) region play a more essential support role than the muscles. They're strong, and outside of severe traumatic accidents, they aren't often seriously injured, though they are a part of the standard back-trauma diagnosis. The muscles of the lumbar spine, on the other hand, are prone to fatigue and shutting down when the system is out of balance. Posture and work habits are key here. If you're spending too much time immobile, sitting or standing, and the forces of gravity aren't being evenly distributed through the soft tissue and the spinal hardware, you're likely to have problems. As we dis-

IMMEDIATE TREATMENT/
WHEN TO SEE A DOCTOR

Any injury or trauma in the vicinity of the spinal cord must be considered serious until proven otherwise. You need to rule out damage to the nerves or to the structures of the spinal column, including the vertebrae, the spinal cord, the spinal ligaments, and the disks. If you have any numbness or loss of sensation or progressive muscle weakness in any part of your body, or a change in your bowel or bladder function, get medical help right away. As with any joint problem, check for any signs of infection such as redness or heat or fever. If there are any, see a doctor immediately. Back pain by itself is not so serious, although it can be excruciating. In most cases, it resolves in a week or two. You may wish to work with a doctor, chiropractor, or muscle therapist to relieve the pain. If the pain lasts longer than a week or two, you certainly should.

cussed in chapter 4, emotional stress often plays a role, as do out-of-the-ordinary activities that jolt the system: playing sports you haven't properly conditioned for, carrying a suitcase on vacation, lifting heavy boxes during a house move.

The good news is that lower-back pain rooted in overtaxed muscles is usually not constant. It comes and goes, sometimes mysteriously. The better news—and it probably is news to a lot of readers—is that manual muscle therapy followed by physical therapy is an extremely effective course of treatment for most garden-variety lower-back pain. Furthermore, as muscle problems can cause spinal dysfunction and restrictions, the combination of manual therapy to address the muscle and chiropractic to realign the spine is also a valuable treatment package. That is where our emphasis lies in this chapter—on the "common backache" and not on the much less frequent cases of structural damage that may require surgery. (Every hot spot tells its own story. Some of the most common knee problems, by comparison, involve joint damage that often requires surgery.)

COMMON PROBLEMS AND CULPRITS

The erector spinae (spinal erectors) climb up the entire length of your back and are the longest muscle group in the body. When both sides of the erector spinae work together, they extend the spine from the cervical to the lumbar region, bringing the head and neck back into extension, straightening the middle (thoracic) spine, and arching the lower back. They also work eccentrically to control the spine as you bend forward. Along with the quadratus lumborum muscles, which lie underneath, the erector spinae work unilaterally to bend and twist the torso. Deepest of all are a group of small muscles, notably the multifii, that support and stabilize your lower and midback. (You strengthen those muscles when you do push-ups or abdominal plank exercises, for example.)

The muscles of the lower back are balanced by the muscles of the front of the trunk—agonist and antagonist. The more important role of the abdominals is not to flex the trunk but to act as a spinal stabilizer and rotator. The rectus abdominis, which flexes and stabilizes, runs straight up from the pubic bone to the rib cage. (It's divided into segments that are visible if you're especially fit and lean—the "washboard abs" look.) The external obliques run diagonally to either side of the rectus abdominis. Assisted by the internal obliques, which run diagonally beneath them, these muscles flex the trunk and aid in side-to-side and twisting movement, as well as supplying core support. The transversus abdominis muscle is the deepest muscle of all. It acts like a girdle of support and assists in breathing.

All of the muscles of the lumbar spine are considered "postural." They're constantly firing in small, subtle ways to maintain the proper alignment of the spine. When the iliopsoas, a powerful muscle group that flexes the hip and the trunk, tightens up, it can pull the spine forward. The erector spinae and core muscles are forced to overwork to maintain the position of the spine, leading to back pain and spasms, which can refer pain away from the area.

WHAT GOES WRONG, AND HOW TO FIX IT

Mostly Muscular

Chronic Lower-Back Pain
Dr. Ted Schwartz, a forty-year-old neurosurgeon at Manhattan's prestigious New York Presbyterian Hospital, had endured chronic back pain since he was in medi-

cal school. He'd studied his own MRI and could see nothing about the structure of his lumbar spine that looked unusual. He wasn't even a candidate for an anti-inflammatory injection near a disk, much less the spinal-fusion operation (removing a damaged disk and fusing the vertebrae together) that he had performed on hundreds of his patients. Dr. Schwartz assumed the problem was mostly muscular, but nothing in his surgeon's toolbox seemed to fit the situation, and his sporadic attempts to address it with back-stretching exercises had gone nowhere. Meanwhile, standing in the operating room for hours on end had become so painful, it threatened to short-circuit his surgical career. "I've always been very skeptical of any nontraditional treatments for back pain," he says, "but I didn't have a lot of good options." After three twenty-minute manual therapy treatments over two weeks, Dr. Schwartz was out of the woods. "That was three years ago, and my back pain hasn't been bad on a chronic basis since," he says. "Now I stretch every morning, and if I get a flare-up, I'll take Aleve." Regarding the treatment itself—Dr. DeStefano manu-

SELF-DEFENSE

PROTECT YOUR LOWER BACK

Don't lean forward from the hips and lock your knees when you're doing standing activities such as washing dishes, vacuuming, shaving, etc.

Avoid twisting your trunk around when you're bending and lifting, such as when unloading laundry or reaching for something in the backseat of a car. Whenever possible, turn your entire body around, and avoid lifting with your back muscles.

When you're lifting heavy objects, lift with the hips and legs, not the back. Keep your back straight, bend at the knees, and keep the heavy object centered and close to your body.

Avoid carrying suitcases or heavy shoulder bags, which stress one side of the back. Rolling suitcases and backpacks are the way to go.

Don't drive in a stretched-out position with your seat reclined. Sit straight and tall—you shouldn't have to reach for the steering wheel. On long car trips, take rest/stretch breaks.

On plane, train, or bus trips, pack a small pillow or rolled-up towel to place behind your lumbar spine or neck.

ally released tightness in the abdominal muscles and the psoas muscle in the front of the trunk and the erector spinae muscles in the lower back—Dr. Schwartz is grateful but not all that curious. "If it worked, it worked," he says. "To this day, I'm not sure I can explain why."

Picture the spine as the mast of a sailing boat stabilized and balanced by wire stays. The wires in the rear of the mast are the back muscles, the erector spinae group. The opposing set of wires in front are the abdominal muscles and the psoas. Remember that muscles, or muscle groups, have to work together: an agonist fires as an antagonist relaxes. For you to bend backward at the waist or move your trunk side to side, those ab and psoas muscles have to lengthen and the back muscles have to contract. To come back to neutral or to lean forward, it's the reverse. If any of these muscles are fatigued and not properly responding, your sailboat mast, or spine, will be out of balance and you're going to feel it. Yet all too often in the treatment of lower-back pain, the front muscles are ignored. The attitude is "Hey, you've got back pain; let's get to work on those back muscles!"

Why Ted Schwartz was more vulnerable to back pain than most of his colleagues, neither he nor we know. But the hours of unrelieved standing had chronically irritated and fatigued the back muscles. Sitting glued to your office chair at work can be just as harmful in a more insidious way. (See the box below on making your office more back-friendly.) Over time, the sitter settles into a rounded-shoulder, slumped-forward position in the chair. The muscles in the front of the torso, espe-

SELF-
DEFENSE

ERGONOMIC/WORK TIPS

Don't stay in the same sitting or standing position for long periods. Take short, frequent breaks to get the circulation and the muscles moving.

Don't lean forward in the chair when you write or work. You may need to pull your chair closer to the desk or the computer or to use a movable keyboard tray. Set up your workspace to minimize having to lean and twist around to do routine tasks.

A good office chair should have armrests and an adjustable lumbar support. Your lower back should be in contact with the back of the chair. The chair should support the natural curve of your lower back, minimizing pressure on muscles and vertebral disks.

cially the psoas, shorten and tighten. This exerts a forward pull on the lumbar spine. To maintain the spine's normal up-and-down alignment, the erector spinae muscles have to pull back, firing constantly, which drives them into fatigue and painful contraction. It's a perpetual tug-of-war in which both sides lose and the person whose body is the battlefield is saddled with lower-back pain. Treatment is straightforward: manually loosening the psoas and the abdominal muscles in the front, taking pressure off the back, then addressing the secondary damage created in the back.

Muscle or Joint?

Traumatic Lower-Back Pain
Holly, a young woman in her midtwenties, had no history of lower-back pain. She was helping her boyfriend install an air conditioner in their house when she felt a sharp, stabbing pain in her lower back and shooting pains running down her leg, the classic sign of a vertebral disk pressing down on the sciatic nerve or "sciatica." Over the next week the pain worsened. Following her primary-care physician's lead, she saw an orthopedic surgeon, who suggested some conservative chiropractic care with muscle work. She improved and her symptoms subsided.

Nowhere in the body is it harder to tease out muscular problems from joint damage than in the spine. Even in cases where the muscle is clearly the bad actor and no structural damage shows up on the MRI, something about the spinal architecture probably makes the affected muscle a little more susceptible. In Holly's case, she does have evidence of joint damage in the form of a mildly herniated disk. But that doesn't mean surgery to remove it is the best course of action. It's possible that an irritated, contracted muscle in the hip rotators may have entrapped the sciatic nerve and caused the shooting or "radicular" pain down the leg. In other words, Holly's damaged disk may be old business and unrelated to the ill-advised air-conditioner lift. Or it could have been a contributing factor, an extra measure of instability in the lumbar region that pushed her overtaxed muscles over the edge. The best and most conservative first line of action would be manual therapy, not only to relieve pain but also to rule out serious disk damage. Even if Holly's disk herniation was the direct result of her recent back trauma, relaxing the muscles around the disk might take enough pressure off it to stop the pain.

Holly had been given the standard back-trauma diagnosis of "sprain/strain"—

back ligaments sprained, back muscles strained. Serious back-ligament sprains are notoriously hard to treat. Fortunately, her problems were mostly muscular. Dr. DeStefano found that she had strained her psoas by lifting the air conditioner in an awkward, bent-over position. In other words, she had the traumatic version of the backache to which office workers are prone—the erector spinae muscles were in pain from the constant effort of countering the forward tug of the psoas. Not only that, but a small hip muscle, the piriformis, had tightened up and clamped down around her sciatic nerve, sending the shooting pains down the leg. If the disk was involved in any of this unhappiness, it wasn't the main player. After several manual therapy treatments, Holly was out of pain.

Chronic Lower-Back Disk Pain

Robert, in his midfifties, is a music-industry producer in Manhattan who had chronic lower-back pain, including radicular pain down one leg. Dr. DeStefano applied chiropractic manipulations along with manual therapy on his muscles, but the progress wasn't good enough. The muscles would relax when they were manually treated, then tighten up again shortly afterward. This was a strong indication that the muscles were irritated by signals sent by a damaged disk, likely the primary source of the problem. Dr. DeStefano referred Robert to Dr. Jennifer Solomon at the Hospital for Special Surgery, who is a physiatrist specializing in the spine and sports medicine. She gave him a single injection of an anti-inflammatory corticosteroid, which quieted down the inflamed nerves and cut his pain by 90 percent. Then Robert returned to Dr. DeStefano to continue the manual therapy. When the muscles of his lower back and front trunk were firing properly and the tissue felt supple and relaxed to the touch, Robert graduated to a physical therapy program. The goal is for him is to leave PT with a handful of stretching and strength exercises that he can do daily or several times a week to keep the muscles in his midsection moving and to minimize the chance that his damaged disk will cause more trouble.

As you've probably gathered by now, the lower back can be a minefield. All the major components—the nerves that branch off from the spinal cord, the cartilage disks that protect the spine, and the postural muscles that support it—work together in proximity. When they get in each other's way, inflammation, irritation, and pain result. But as Robert's case shows, even when the disk is the primary problem, it doesn't necessarily follow that surgery is always the best treatment. In our experi-

CORTICOSTEROID INJECTIONS

An injection of a corticosteroid around a nerve or in a joint reduces local inflammation, which gives the area a break from irritation and the chance to heal. Drugs such as cortisone and prednisone are similar to the steroid hormones your own body produces. When conservative measures such as chiropractic and muscle therapy aren't enough by themselves, the corticosteroids can be a useful addition to the treatment toolbox, but if they're overused, they can damage tendons and ligaments. No more than three injections in a given area over a year is the usual rule of thumb.

ence, the best orthopedic surgeons are cautious about operating on disks. But as our colleague Dr. Solomon says, "I have patients who come into my office who will never get better because they're convinced that surgery is the answer to all their back problems." We subscribe to what Dr. Solomon calls a "big-picture approach" to the spine: chiropractic, muscle therapy to address muscular tightness, physical therapy to retrain posture and movement, and, when necessary, medical or surgical intervention. With Robert and other patients, she's had excellent success treating them with a single corticosteroid injection to break the chronic-pain cycle and give the body a chance to heal.

Joint/Orthopedic

Lower-Back Disk Pain (with Severe Neurological Symptoms)
If the nerve pain that radiates down through the body is severe and unrelenting and the muscles connected to those nerves are getting progressively weaker, medical attention is crucial, and surgery is likely your best option.

Facet Joint Syndrome
Branching off each pair of vertebrae are small protrusions, the facets, which form joints with the facets above and below them. They help stabilize the vertebrae and allow for a limited amount of movement. And just like the knee or the hip, the facet

joints can wear out, becoming one source of persistent back pain in older people. The disks, the shock absorbers between the vertebrae, shrink with age, increasing the pressure on the facets and the likelihood that cartilage will wear away and bone will wind up grinding against bone—possibly causing arthritis.

Surgery to fuse the vertebrae and the facets is one treatment option that, when necessary, has good results. Patients are usually older, however, and may not tolerate the considerable risks of the operation. Whenever possible, we take the most conservative approach, focusing on the things we do for patients (manual therapy for muscle tightness; corticosteroid injections if necessary) and things patients must do for themselves (losing weight to take pressure off the lumbar spine; going to physical therapy and incorporating PT exercises into a daily routine; getting the body moving in a low-impact way with walking, aqua exercises, or cycling).

Spinal Stenosis

Like arthritis, spinal stenosis is a structural problem that doesn't usually have a good structural solution. The spine changes with age—the vertebrae can develop bone spurs, disks can bulge—which can narrow the space inside the spinal column through which the nerve fibers travel. When the fit is so tight that the nerve fibers get compressed, the diagnosis is spinal stenosis. The symptoms are muscle pain and weakness, sometimes accompanied by numbness and tingling. Patients are usually seniors, who are not good candidates for surgery to open up the spinal canal. Sometimes treating the symptoms can eliminate pain for patients who cannot tolerate surgery.

Our point is that diagnoses such as facet-joint arthritis and spinal stenosis aren't, or shouldn't be, the last word on what you can and can't do in life. Yes, the ability of your lumbar spine to do its job has been compromised by structural changes inside the joints. So the onus is on you to get more out of the function you do have by addressing muscle strength, weight control, and exercise. We have a patient, a ninety-two-year-old gentleman, who had been a vigorous long-distance walker all his life until classic spinal stenosis symptoms reduced him to a shuffle. A few sessions of manual muscle therapy had won him only modest gains. The next time we saw him, he had returned from spending the winter in Arizona, where a resourceful physical therapist had worked on strengthening exercises to build up those leg muscles that were still connected to the nerves. He was back up to walking a mile a day. Although his condition wasn't corrected, he had fewer symptoms.

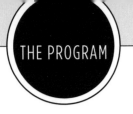

LOWER BACK

The lower back has a complex of muscles that both stabilize the back and create a wide variety of movements. The lower back is affected by all the core muscles, which form a muscular corset around the lower torso and hips. Any imbalance or restriction can put strain on the back muscles and have an adverse affect on posture.

LOWER BACK

Purpose: To target and remove any restrictions and restore a full range of motion to the erector spinae muscles (the main postural muscles of the back) by manually releasing tight, short, and damaged muscles.

Starting out: Sit on a stability ball with your feet spread shoulders' width apart. Rotate slightly toward the treatment side and arch your back. Grip a F.A.S.T. Stick™ or other treatment stick, such as a TheraCane®, behind the back, with both palms facing forward, and place the knob on the thick muscle on the treatment side of your spine. This muscle is divided into three zones: zone one is closest to the spine, zone two is in the middle of that thick muscle, and zone three is on the outside edge of this large muscle group.

How to do it: Press in and down slightly, as though trying to slide the muscle down the back. Keeping the stick's pressure constant, bend forward and rotate away from the treatment side as far as is pain- and strain-free. Repeat on the opposite side. Do two to three passes, releasing and moving the stick position each time from the hips toward the midback in each zone.

Troubleshooting: Don't press too hard as this can irritate the muscle. Do not place the stick on bone. Avoid letting the skin slide under the stick—make sure the stick moves with the body.

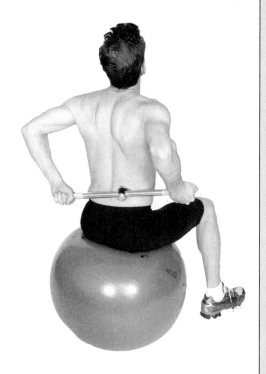

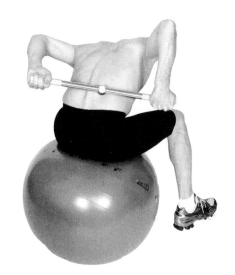

LATERAL LOWER BACK

A. ANTERIOR QUADRATUS LUMBORUM

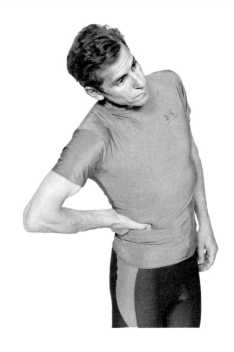

Purpose: To target and remove any restrictions and restore a full range of motion in the anterior lateral fibers of the quadratus lumborum muscle by manually releasing tight, short, and damaged muscles. This muscle affects both the lower back and the gait cycle.

Starting out: Stand with your feet spread shoulders' width apart. Bend toward the treatment side, without bending forward or back. Relax the muscles and place your hand around the side just below the ribs, with the thumb to the front and the fingers to the back. You should feel the hip bone at the webbing of the thumb, then move up approximately one inch onto the muscle.

How to do it: Press in and slightly down with the thumb—think of hooking the thumb around the muscle. Keeping a steady hold so the skin does not slide and your hand stays in position, laterally bend to the opposite side. Do two to three passes, releasing and replacing your hand each time. Repeat on the other side.

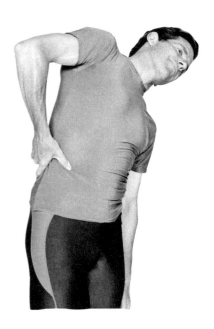

Troubleshooting: Don't press too hard too fast; let the hand "sink in." Avoid letting the skin slide under the hand by using angled pressure. Don't collapse to the side; keep tall in the torso as you bend to either side. Don't press directly on the hip bone or the ribs.

B. POSTERIOR QUADRATUS LUMBORUM

Purpose: To target and remove any restrictions and restore a full range of motion to the posterior lateral fibers of the quadratus lumborum muscle by manually releasing tight, short, and damaged muscles. This muscle affects both the back and the gait cycle.

Starting out: Stand with your feet spread shoulders' width apart. Bend your body toward the treatment side, without bending forward or back. Relax the muscles and place your hand around the side just below the ribs, with your fingers to the front and the thumb to the back. You should feel the hip bone at the edge of your palm, then move up approximately one inch onto the muscle.

How to do it: Press in and down with the thumb and pull the muscle on the front with your fingers. Keeping a steady grip so the skin does not slide and the hand stays in position, bend your torso to the opposite side. Do two to three passes, releasing and replacing the hand a little higher each time. Repeat on the other side.

Troubleshooting: Don't press too hard too fast; let your hand "sink in." Avoid letting the skin slide under your hand by using angled pressure. Don't collapse to the side; stand erect without flexing forward or back as you bend to either side.

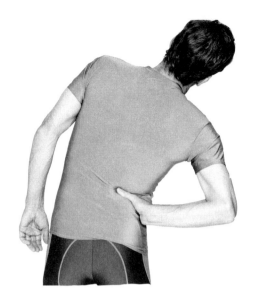

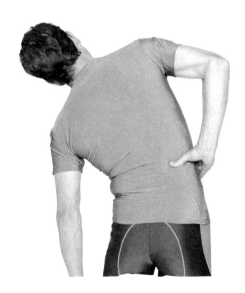

ABDOMEN (ANTERIOR LOWER BACK)

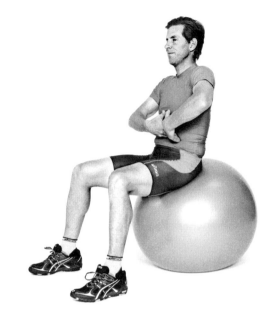

Purpose: To target and remove any restrictions and restore a full range of motion to the abdominal muscles and fascia by manually releasing tight, short, and damaged muscles. These muscles affect both posture and balance and innumerable movements.

Starting out: Sit on a stability ball with your feet spread a little wider than shoulders' width apart. Relax your abdominals and touch your belly with your hands: fingers flat, one hand over the other with the fingertips lined up, palms in. The abdominals should be divided into two zones from the ribs to the hip/pubic bones. Zone one is to the right of the belly button, zone two is to the left of the belly button.

How to do it: Once contact is made, press in and up toward the ribs with your fingers. Keeping a steady grip so the skin does not slide and you do not lose your placement, lean back onto the ball. Do two to three passes in each zone, releasing and moving the hands closer to the ribs each time. Note: tension can also be in and down toward feet during treatment. Try both directions to see which feels better.

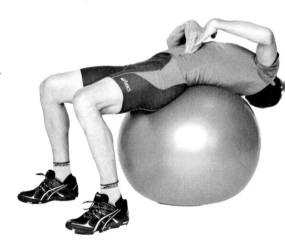

As an alternative, do this self-treatment on the floor, following the same protocol as above.

Troubleshooting: Don't press too hard too fast; let the hand "sink in." Keep your pressure down toward the knees or up toward the ribs, not straight into the belly. Stay "long" in the torso as you control the motion up and down—let the ball support you.

LOWER BACK

A. KNEES TO CHEST

Purpose: To lengthen the muscles of the lower back and the muscle junction of the lower back and hips. This can be a valuable morning stretch for those who wake up with a stiff back.

Starting out: Lie on your back with both knees bent and hips' width apart. Both feet should be flat on the floor, or the legs can be extended if that is comfortable.

How to do it: Grip one leg with both hands placed just below the kneecap and bring the knee to the chest slowly and only as far as there is no pain (either in the hip or back). If this motion is comfortable on both sides individually, try both legs together. Put one hand around each knee just below the kneecap and bring both knees simultaneously to the chest in a pain-free range of motion. The stretch should be held for two seconds, then return to the starting position. Repeat ten times.

Troubleshooting: Don't allow the knees to fall out to the side, or the hips to come off the floor. Allow the upper back and head to stay relaxed. When using both legs, keep the spine as flat on the floor as possible, so the body does not rock back and forth. Only your hips should come off the floor. If you can't reach your knees comfortably, a strap can be used to bring the knees to the chest so that your head and back can stay on the floor.

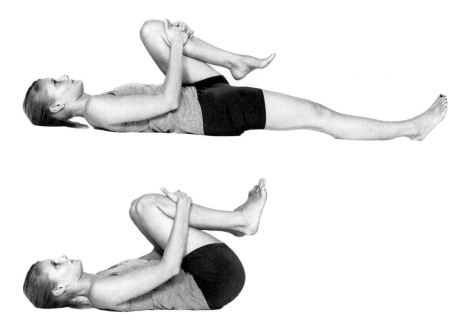

B. CORE BALL STRETCH

Purpose: To lengthen the muscles of the lower back and their junction with the muscles of the hip. This stretch also creates a gentle traction on the spine and so lengthens the smaller, intrinsic spinal muscles.

Starting out: Kneel in front of a stability ball with hands and upper body partially on the ball.

How to do it: Allow your weight to transfer to the ball, slowly rolling your chest, then abdomen, onto the ball, until your hands reach the floor and only your toes remain on the floor on the other side. Relinquish all of your body weight into the ball; you should feel a gentle traction in the lower back. Hold the stretch for two seconds, then return to the starting position. Repeat ten times.

Troubleshooting: Keep your feet and hands wide enough so that you feel stable on the ball. Allow your upper back and head to stay relaxed. The stretch should feel gentle, so only roll onto the ball as far as is comfortable.

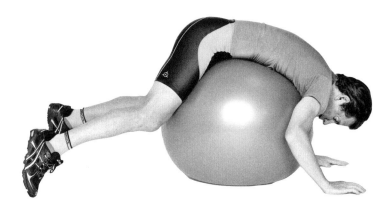

C. CAT/COW

Purpose: To lengthen the muscles of the core. This is a more active stretch that further mobilizes the vertebrae, warms up the muscles, and helps to increase range of motion.

Starting out: Start on all fours with a comfortable, neutral spine. Your head should be in line with the spine, and you should be looking straight down.

How to do it: Begin by arching your back, gently pushing your belly forward, lifting your head, and looking up, while allowing your abdomen to relax. Hold the stretch for two to three seconds, then return to the starting position. Round your back as though trying to touch your midback to the ceiling. Then, tuck your hips under and contract your abs. If this is comfortable, you can then tuck your chin as though holding a tennis ball. Hold for two to three seconds, then return to the starting position. Repeat the two stretches ten times.

Troubleshooting: Keep a relaxed neck—do not crunch it back or forward. Keep your feet and hands wide enough so that you feel stable. The stretch should feel gentle, so only curve your spine as much as is comfortable. Keep your knees under your hips, and your hands and elbows under your shoulders.

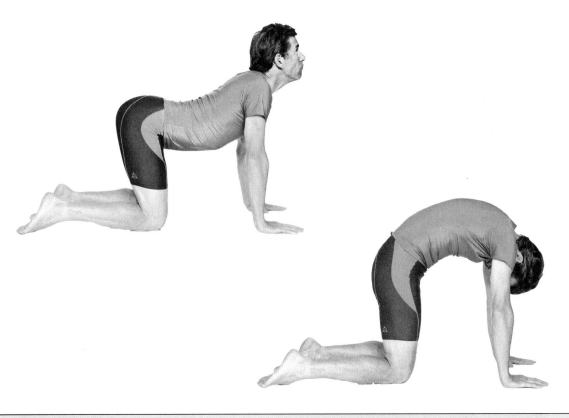

LATERAL LOWER BACK

Purpose: To lengthen the muscles and fascia of the lateral core. Complementing the stretches on the previous page with this side stretch is a great way to mobilize the spine.

Starting out: Standing, bend toward one side with the arm on that side outstretched. Keep your other arm bent at the elbow, and the hand on your hip.

How to do it: Laterally flex toward the opposite side, reaching the outstretched arm over your head. Keep your other hand on your hip for stability.

For an advanced stretch, try dropping the hand from the hip, and reaching as far down the leg as you can, while continuing to reach overhead with the opposite hand.

Troubleshooting: Keep your feet wide enough to feel stable. For additional stretch options, you can lean slightly forward or back as you laterally bend. Do not lean far enough in either direction to cause strain to the back.

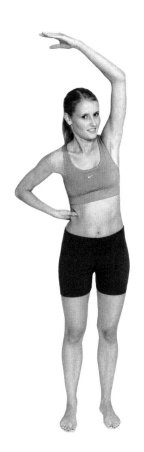

ABDOMEN (ANTERIOR LOWER BACK)

Purpose: To lengthen the abdominals and hip flexors and relax the muscles of the back. A tight abdomen and hips can negatively affect the back and posture. Complementing this stretch with the stretches on the previous pages is a great way to mobilize the spine.

Starting out: Sit on a stability ball and roll your back onto it so that the ball supports your back. Your hands are either out to your sides for balance or over your head to increase the stretch. Your knees should be bent to 90 degrees and your body relaxed and balanced.

How to do it: Allow your weight to transfer from your feet to the ball, slowly rolling the lower back farther onto the ball by extending your knees. Your arms can be extended farther overhead if you can easily keep balance. Hold the stretch for two to three seconds, then return to the starting position. Repeat ten times.

Troubleshooting: Keep your feet and hands wide enough so that you feel stable on the ball. Keep your upper back and head relaxed. The stretch should feel gentle, so only roll onto the ball as far as is comfortable. Keep your feet flat on the floor for stability.

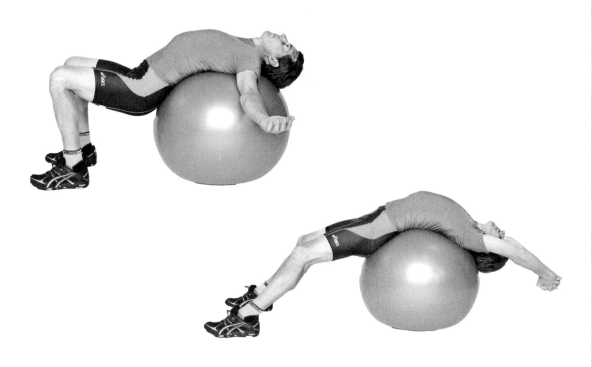

LOWER BACK

SUPERMAN

Purpose: To strengthen the muscles of the lower back and core and the back of the body in general. This contributes to posture and balance, as well as general spine health.

Starting out: Lie facedown with your feet and legs together, mouth to the ground, neutral spine, and arms out to your sides, with hands at hip level.

How to do it: Squeeze your glutes and legs together and stabilize by contracting your abdominals. Then squeeze the shoulder blades together and lift your arms, upper back, and head off the floor. Hold for a count of two. Do ten repetitions, held for no more than two seconds each.

Advanced variation: All is the same except for the arm position. Start with the arms at a right angle from the torso, with the thumbs sticking up. Keep the arms in this position as they are lifted off the floor thumb first.

Troubleshooting: Do not release the stabilizing contraction of your lower and middle body. Keep looking at the floor and relax your head. Remember to breathe and don't clench your teeth.

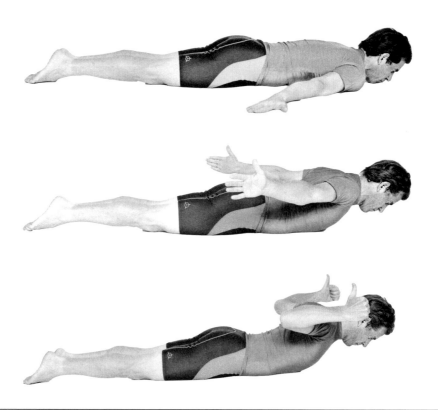

LATERAL LOWER BACK

SIDE PLANK

Purpose: To strengthen the quadratus lumborum, the muscles of the lateral torso, and the core in general. This contributes to posture, balance, and gait, as well as general spine health. This will also warm up the muscles and help prevent strain on other structures.

Starting out: Start on your side, on your hip, knee, and elbow. The elbow should be directly under the shoulder, and the knee should be bent to ninety degrees and in line with the body.

How to do it: Squeeze your glutes and legs together and stabilize by contracting your abdominals and shoulder blades. Lift your hips off the floor and hold the body in a straight line while slowly exhaling. Hold for a count of two. Repeat on the opposite side. Do ten repetitions, held for no more than two seconds each.

Advanced variation: All is the same, except you start with your legs extended straight out and in line with the body. The motion is done the same way, except your weight rests on the side of the bottom foot instead of the knee. You may want to try this with shoes on.

Troubleshooting: Do not release the stabilizing contraction of your lower and middle body and arms. Keep looking straight ahead and keep your neck in line with the spine and relaxed. Remember to breathe and don't clench your teeth. Return to the starting position in a slow and controlled manner.

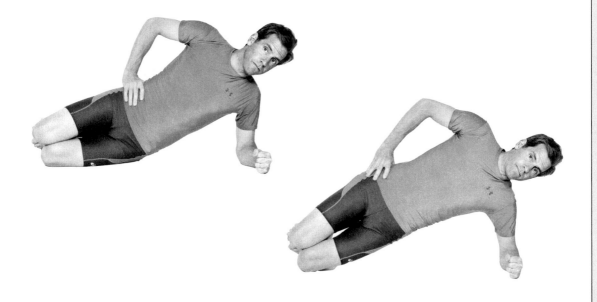

ABDOMEN (ANTERIOR LOWER BACK)

A. PLANK

Purpose: To strengthen the muscles of the core in general. This contributes to posture and balance, as well as general spine health. This will also warm up the muscles and help prevent strain on other structures.

Starting out: Start on your elbows and knees: your elbows should be directly under your shoulders, and your knees should be behind your hips about a hand's length. Your neck should be neutral with your eyes on the floor.

How to do it: Squeeze your glutes and legs together and stabilize by contracting your abdominals and shoulder blades. Lift your knees off the floor and hold your body in a straight line while slowly exhaling. Adjust your foot position so your body is completely straight (without your butt sticking up). Hold this for a count of two. Do ten repetitions, held for no more than two seconds each.

Troubleshooting: Do not release the stabilizing contraction of your lower and middle body and arms. Keep your eyes on the floor and your head relaxed. Remember to breathe and don't clench your teeth. Return to the starting position in a slow and controlled manner.

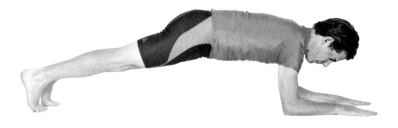

B. STABILITY-BALL CRUNCH

Purpose: To strengthen the abdominals and the core in general. This contributes to posture and balance, as well as general spine health. This will also warm up the muscles and help prevent strain on other structures of the upper body.

Starting out: Sit on a stability ball and roll your back onto it so that the ball supports your back and your knees are bent to 90 degrees. Your feet should be placed as wide as they need to be for balance.

How to do it: Place your hands loosely at ear level, squeeze your glutes and legs, and stabilize by contracting your abdominals and shoulder blades. With a straight back, slowly contract your abs and lift yourself off the ball, only coming up as far as you can without pain. If good form can't be maintained, don't come up as far. Hold for a count of two, slowly release the abs and glutes, and return to the starting position. Do ten repetitions, held for no more than two seconds each.

Troubleshooting: Do not release the stabilizing contraction of your lower and middle body. Keep your neck relaxed and neutral. Remember to breathe and don't clench your teeth. Do not round your back—keep it straight throughout the movement. If you have any neck or back issues, or trouble balancing, see the sit-up alternative on page 59.

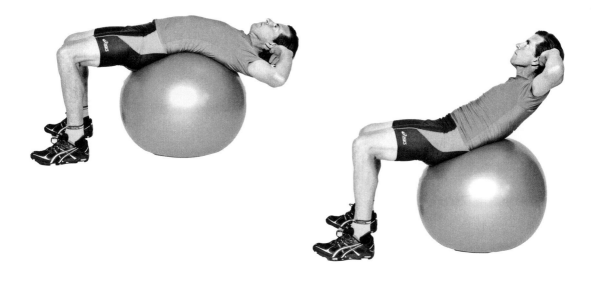

FULL BODY/CORE

A. BALL BOUNCE

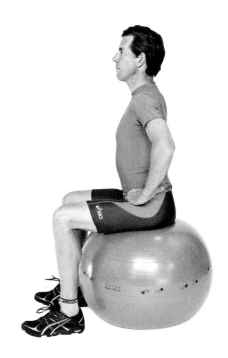

Purpose: To strengthen the muscles of the core in general. This contributes to posture and balance, as well as general spine health. This will also warm up the muscles and help prevent strain on other structures of the upper body.

Starting out: Sit on a stability ball with your feet and knees shoulders' width apart and your knees at a right angle. Observe an upright but relaxed posture.

How to do it: Begin by squeezing your glutes and legs together and contracting the abdominals. This contraction, followed by a slight release, should create a gentle bouncing motion. Do ten repetitions, then build up to more as you get stronger.

Troubleshooting: Look straight and keep your head relaxed. Remember to breathe and to not lean forward or back.

B. SINGLE-LEG TOE TOUCH

Purpose: To strengthen the muscles of the core and body as they contribute to balance and stabilization.

Starting out: Stand balanced on one foot, keeping your back and neck in a straight line. Keep your eyes fixed on a point on the floor about four feet in front of your foot.

How to do it: Keeping your eyes fixed on that point, hinge at the waist and reach your opposite hand to touch the supporting foot. Hold for a count of two. Repeat with the opposite hand and foot. Do ten repetitions, without stopping if possible.

Troubleshooting: Move slowly and maintain a stable balance. Bend the knee as much as necessary to balance and stay pain-free. The goal is not to reach the foot but to stay steady, so focus on relaxed stability and not on the distance between your hand and foot. Keep your eyes fixed on a point, and your head relaxed. Remember to breathe and don't clench the teeth.

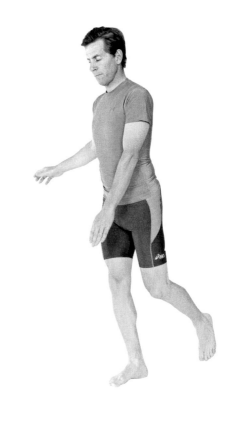

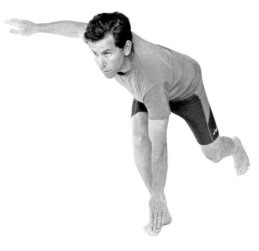

C. KETTLE BELL SWING

Purpose: To strengthen the muscles of the core and the rest of body as they pertain to balance and safe back movement.

Starting out: Stand straight up with your feet slightly wider than shoulders' width apart and hold a kettle bell with both hands at the midline.

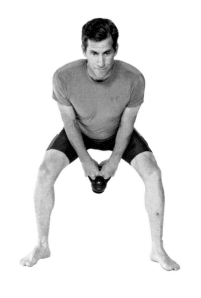

How to do it: Stabilize by contracting your abdominals and shoulder blades. Keeping a flat back, bend your knees and bend forward at the waist to swing the kettle bell through your legs. Then contract the abs, glutes, and legs together with your shoulders and back to swing the kettle bell up to forehead level or higher as you straighten your knees. Keep the motion continuous. The object is to use all the core muscles to control the weight and keep it swinging smoothly. Do ten repetitions. If a kettle bell is not available, any weight (dumbbell, can of soup) can be used as long as it is held firmly.

Troubleshooting: Look straight and keep your head relaxed. Remember to breathe and don't clench your teeth. Don't lock your knees or let the kettle bell swing out of control. This should be a controlled, rhythmic swing, where the body works with the momentum of the weight. If you have back pain or previous back issues, check with a physician or therapist before attempting this exercise.

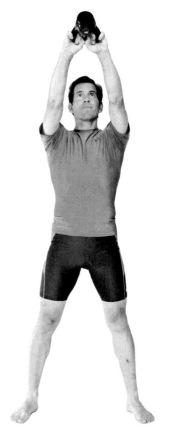

THE HIP

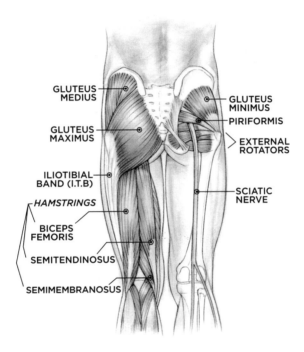

GLUTEUS MEDIUS

GLUTEUS MAXIMUS

ILIOTIBIAL BAND (I.T.B)

HAMSTRINGS

BICEPS FEMORIS

SEMITENDINOSUS

SEMIMEMBRANOSUS

GLUTEUS MINIMUS

PIRIFORMIS

EXTERNAL ROTATORS

SCIATIC NERVE

INTRODUCING THE HIP

The hip can be a puzzle. An injury here can show up as muscle pain in the thigh or the butt, or a strain in the lower-back or abdominal area. What makes the hip a difficult joint to diagnose is its design. For the system to work the way it's supposed to, not only does the joint have to move without a serious hitch, but the twenty-seven muscles that cross the hip also have to fire in perfect synchrony.

Yet the hip looks so stable, orthopedists have only recently begun to see it as a likely suspect behind midsection pain that was typically blamed on the lower back or else shrugged off as "only muscular." The hip joint is where the thighbone (femur) joins the girdle of three bones called the pelvis.

The design of the hip joint is a true ball-in-socket: the ball-shaped protuberance at the top of the thighbone (or femur) fits into the hip socket (or acetabulum) of the pelvis. The acetabulum is lined with a ring of fibrous cartilage called the labrum that helps hold the "ball" in place, and an intracapsular ligament connects the ball to the socket. Surrounding the joint is a sleeve of collagen known as the capsule, which is reinforced by several thickenings within the capsular structure known as extracapsular ligaments.

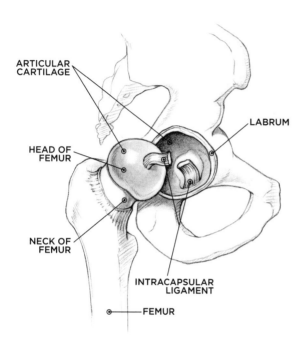

ARTICULAR CARTILAGE

LABRUM

HEAD OF FEMUR

NECK OF FEMUR

INTRACAPSULAR LIGAMENT

FEMUR

Looking at the hip as an integrated system of muscle, joint, and bone has, over the past decade, changed the way the top specialists diagnose and treat it. Two questions in particular troubled doctors. Why were so many well-conditioned athletes straining or tearing their abdominal and adductor (inner-thigh) muscles, the so-called sports hernia? Why were so many older people losing their hip function to osteoarthritis and needing hip replacement surgery? One's a muscle problem, one's a bone problem, and yet there was an emerging common link: what happens inside the hip joint. A recently appreciated source of hip pain is called femoroacetabular impingement. The ball of the femur can't move around properly because of bony bumps on the femoral ball, or friction against the hip socket. This alters the way the body's entire midsection moves, straining the abdominal and the adductor muscles, making them vulnerable to tearing. Over time, an impinged hip can tear the supporting labrum, which can lead to bone-on-bone friction, then to arthritis, which can eventually result in a hip replacement.

IMMEDIATE TREATMENT/
WHEN TO SEE A DOCTOR

The hip is a sturdy joint, so if you feel a sudden pop or experience the onset of sudden severe pain, it could be something serious such as a tendon or a labrum tear. See a doctor sooner rather than later. It usually takes a severe trauma such as a high-speed car accident to dislocate the hip (where the femur comes out of the hip socket), so if that happens, you'll find yourself in the emergency room anyway. As with any joint problem, check for any signs of infection—redness, heat or fever, pain not connected to changes in activity. If there are any, see a doctor immediately. When the dire possibilities have been ruled out, you can assume you've got some kind of soft-tissue damage, usually a muscle or joint strain or sprain. The normal rules of RICE apply: Rest (keep weight off the area); Ice it; keep inflammation down with Compression (a compression bandage or bike shorts, which can contain the ice); and Elevation (bring the affected area above the level of your heart). It's your call whether you want to seek out a doctor or muscle therapist right away, but if you still can't put weight on your leg after one or two weeks, it's time.

Combining the most advanced orthopedic surgical procedures with the most effective manual therapeutic techniques, we have created a state-of-the-art approach for dealing with the entire range of hip problems. These include the problems that require surgery (and receive muscle work before and after), and the ones that can successfully be treated, and self-treated, by working on the muscles only—no scalpel or arthroscope required.

WHAT GOES WRONG, AND HOW TO FIX IT

Mostly Muscular

Groin Pain

Amy is a successful, disciplined Manhattan woman in her early thirties who works in the financial industry. She takes her running seriously. But for the past several months, she's been bothered by groin pain when she runs. She tried to run through

COMMON PROBLEMS AND CULPRITS

The iliopsoas and the rectus femoris are two muscles that flex the hip exclusively, bringing the thigh up toward the torso. The rectus femoris is a big, visible muscle that gives definition to the front of the thigh. But the ropy iliopsoas (actually, three muscles that merge: the psoas major and minor and the iliacus; see page 197), buried deep in the pelvic region, is the more common troublemaker. The psoas major originates on the lower third of the spine and runs from the front of the spine to just inside the top of the femur, or thighbone, in the groin area. If it tightens up, it can painfully press against the hip capsule, which protects the hip joint, causing front-of-the-hip pain. If the iliopsoas fatigues and shuts down, it forces the rectus femoris to overwork, causing front-of-the-hip thigh soreness and irritation. Or it can shorten and pull the spinal column forward, forcing the back muscles to constantly pull back to keep the spine straight. The result: lower-back spasm and pain.

The seven adductor muscles of the inner thigh bring the leg toward the center of the body and also help with stabilization. The kind of lateral motion demanded by such sports as soccer, tennis, basketball, and hockey is tough on the body's lower half. Not only are the adductors prone to strain and tear (so-called groin pulls), causing soreness in the groin area, but a major abdominal muscle, the rectus abdominis, can strain at the same time. Then you've got a more serious, harder-to-heal, and still not entirely understood condition called athletic pubalgia (or sports hernia).

Two versatile muscles that run along the outside of the hip, the gluteus medius and minimus, abduct the leg, that is, they bring the leg out to the side of the body. They too can become strained, causing soreness in the outer-hip area and symptoms that can mimic sciatica. A small neighboring muscle that helps externally rotate the hip, the piriformis, can entrap the sciatic nerve and send pain shooting down the posterior leg. Besides piriformis syndrome, and pseudo-sciatica from the glutes, a number of other less common and often hard-to-diagnose nerve entrapment syndromes in the hip area can deliver pain and numbness to the groin and legs.

The large muscles that cross the hip and the knee from behind are easier to assess. The gluteus maximus is the muscle that gives the buttock its rounded shape. It helps to attach the pelvis to the femur. The hamstrings run down the back of the thigh, connecting the pelvis to the femur and lower leg bones. Together, the gluteus maximus and the hamstrings pull the upper and lower leg backward, the power stroke that assists walking and running. The gluteus maximus is quite resilient and hard to tear. The worst you're likely to get is sore if you overdo running or cycling up hills. That's not the case with the hamstrings, which are probably strained more often than any other muscle group in the body. The hamstrings provide a decelerating force, stopping the hip from over-flexing during the gait cycle, by balancing and controlling the forward pull of the quads. This decelerating force, which involves contraction and lengthening at the same time, is stressful to the muscles fibers and can often result in injury.

the pain, but it only got worse. She went to her internist, who diagnosed a groin pull and sent her to a physical therapist, who helped her to strengthen her core muscles. But that only caused the pain to flare up. Then the internist ordered an MRI of her lumbar spine, which showed a slight bulge in one of the spinal disks, so he sent her to a neurosurgeon. The neurosurgeon didn't think the bulge was all that interesting, so he sent her back to physical therapy to strengthen her back muscles. Finally, the groin pain lessened, and desperate to get back to her running routine, Amy returned to the Central Park Reservoir track. Before she'd finished her first lap, that familiar aching pain returned to her inner thigh.

When you strain a muscle once, the odds are you've simply overdone it. You've asked the muscle to fire too hard or too fast. (RICE should take care of the problem.) When a muscle or a group of muscles strain repeatedly, your body is trying to tell you something. Something about the way the muscles, joints, and bones mesh in movement is setting you up for pain. It could be a problem with your form—something you can change, such as the way you carry your arms or which part of the foot you land on. Or it could be "biomechanical," for instance, the way your hip rotates or your foot turns in when you run.

Amy had something more than a garden-variety groin pull. Both her abdominal and adductor (inner thigh) muscles were severely irritated and fatigued. In the elite male athletes that Dr. Kelly often studies and treats, this syndrome is called athletic pubalgia (or, popularly, the sports hernia), and femoral acetabular impingement, or hip impingement, is an increasingly recognized reason those muscles are under such strain. But Amy's hip didn't look that bad. The problem is that normal running motion creates extra twisting forces in the hip joint when the leg strikes the ground. This occurrence is not as common in men, but women generally have a wider pelvis, creating a greater angle of the femur (in sports medicine lingo, they have a wider "Q angle"), and that puts the abdominal muscles and hip joint under greater tension. For a significant number of women joggers, the abs and the adductors have to work overtime to stabilize the lower back and the hips. The result can be the disabling groin pain that sent Amy on her medical merry-go-round.

So the treatment emphasis was to manually release tension in the abdominals and these two muscle groups of the hip, the adductors and the abductors. (Recall that the abductors primarily bring the leg out to the side; the adductors bring the leg in toward the midline.) After several sessions, the muscle fibers had relaxed and normal blood flow had returned to the area, speeding the body's natural healing. Amy was able to resume running. With the muscle damage repaired, she was able to go through a successful course of physical therapy. Strengthening her core muscles is the best assurance the problem won't return.

Front-of-the-Hip Pain: Hip Flexor Tendinitis

Joe, thirty, was a solid power forward on his high school basketball team, and although he wasn't powerful (or tall or quick) enough to make his college team, he played intramural ball and then rec league hoops when he went to work on Wall Street. One winter, the normally hearty Joe began to suffer twinges of hip pain as he ran up and down the court. At first, only the running irritated the hip, but after a few weeks he felt a jolt of pain in the left hip when he got out of bed in the morning. If he sat too long at work, he had to walk off that achy, cramped feeling. Joe's orthopedist ruled out joint injury and sent him to a physical therapist to address the hip tendinitis. At first, the PT "modalities"—whirlpool, ultrasound, and electrical stimulation—calmed down the inflamed area. But then he felt a familiar tightness when he tried to strengthen the leg on the exercise bike, and a return to the basketball court brought back the old pain.

Joe's story illustrates the importance of the "kinetic chain," the linkage of muscles and joints that allows us to move. When one important link in the chain is damaged, the body has to compensate, and invariably the trouble is passed up or down the line. In Joe's case, the bad link is the iliopsoas group, the muscles buried deep in the pelvic region that pull the thigh up and out. Joe's iliopsoas was so fatigued from his sudden increase in activity, it had practically shut down, shifting the burden of flexing the hip to the rectus femoris, a long muscle that runs down the thigh from the hip bone to the knee. In turn, this thigh muscle became so overwhelmed, it tightened up, tugging against the tendon that attaches it to the hip bone. The problem inflamed the surrounding tissues and hobbled Joe on the basketball court.

Manually treating Joe, Dr. DeStefano worked on the iliopsoas and the rectus femoris and a couple of smaller muscles that help out with hip flexion, in addition to chiropractic treatments. But just as important, he worked with Joe to get at the root of the breakdown. Joe's overall muscular fitness had been in decline since college and had taken a steep dive two years before when he and his wife had a child. Joe still had the self-image of an athlete and enough "game" to be a threat on the court. But without the conditioning base provided by constant physical activity, his muscles had lost the strength and resilience they needed to handle the stress of Joe's jumping from a sedentary lifestyle to his winter regimen of basketball two nights a week. His setup at work did him no favors either. He was always swiveling to the left to answer his phone, which, over time, had tightened up one side of his lumbar spine, an imbalance that contributed to his psoas woes.

After the hip flexors had healed—and the desk was rearranged—Joe went to a talented physical therapist for a couple of weeks of targeted flexibility and strength work. Subsequently, Joe teamed up with a good personal trainer, building enough gym time and all-around conditioning into his busy schedule so that he could hit the basketball court without its hitting back.

Back-of-the-Hip Pain: Hamstrings and Gluteals

Sue, forty, is an executive secretary from New Jersey who never cared much for sports and was happy to do without. But with her weight and her cholesterol numbers steadily creeping upward, her doctor advised her to go on an exercise program. Sue got a gung ho trainer who gave her an aggressive routine of "clamshell" exercises when she told him she wanted more definition in her butt. She was delighted with the results until her butt muscles developed a persistent ache that wouldn't go away even after a few days off from the gym. Instead, the pain traveled partway down the back of her thigh. So much for trying to get in shape, she figured, and returned to the couch.

The muscles behind the hip, the gluteus maximus, which wraps around the buttocks, and the hamstrings, which run down the back of the thighs, are powerhouses. They look bulging and impressive as they power a sprinter or a football running back. But as Sue discovered, the two smaller muscles in the glute family, the gluteus medius and minimus, can be more sensitive and troublesome. Located on the outside of the hip, they're sometimes referred to as the abductors, because they bring the leg out to the side (or abduct). The glute exercises that Sue was assigned can stress these abductors if the intensity is ramped up too quickly. The same thing can happen in yoga or gymnastics. Not only do the muscles become sore and painful, but they can create a condition called pseudo-sciatica, which sends pain down the back of the leg. A little muscle that helps rotate the hip, the piriformis, is actually the most common culprit when it comes to entrapping the sciatic nerve. Piriformis syndrome is a classic "referred pain" syndrome in which the source of the pain (the entrapped sciatic nerve) is sometimes somewhere other than where the pain is felt. When attention is focused on the structures of the lumbar spine, which can cause similar symptoms, or true sciatica, these other conditions are sometimes overlooked.

When Sue's glutes, hamstrings, and hip rotator muscles were manually released, her symptoms resolved. The answer was clear: the butt, not the back, was to blame. Sue returned to an exercise program, this time under the guidance of a personal trainer who subscribed to a "slow and steady" philosophy.

We should add that abductor muscles aren't a problem only for the exercise novice. Running gives runners toned muscles in the front of the thigh (quadriceps) and the back (hamstrings). But if runners or

SELF-DEFENSE

Don't sit in a position where your hips are lower than your knees, either sunk down in a cushy chair or with your legs propped up on a support higher than the chair.

Don't cross your legs. Crossing your legs in a figure 4 position exerts a "twisting out" pressure on the hip. Crossing one thigh over the other exerts a "twisting in" pressure. Both are bad.

Sleeping on your side is, for most people, the healthiest position. Slide a pillow between your knees to relieve the pressure on the hip from the top leg pressing down. This is especially helpful for women with wider Q angles.

If you know you have hip weakness or vulnerability, avoid extreme ranges of movement while symptomatic, as in dance, yoga, or extreme stretching.

joggers don't do anything besides run for exercise, their abductor muscles on the outside of the hip may be so out of balance that they struggle to keep the pelvis level as the legs turn over in the running stride. The stride is therefore less efficient and can lead to injury.

Muscle or Joint?

Groin Pain: Sports Hernia/Hip Impingement

Jane, thirty, is a businesswoman in New Jersey and a promising recreational marathoner. But after her second marathon, she felt as if she weren't the same runner. She had a constant dull ache in her groin area and a propensity to pull a groin muscle every time she stepped up her training. She fit the pattern for sports hernia or athletic pubalgia. Dr. DeStefano would manually treat her abdominal and adductor muscles and win her relief from the pain for a while, then she'd strain another muscle. That suggested that the root problem was the joint, not the muscles. Sure enough, Dr. Kelly ordered an MRI that revealed that her hip joint was too tight and the ring of cartilage that supports it, the labrum, had torn. He made the necessary surgical repairs, and Dr. DeStefano worked on the muscles before and after the operation to speed recovery. Several weeks after the procedure, the hip joint and the muscles that drive it were sufficiently healed that Jane could start physical therapy to build up her core strength and flexibility.

Conventional medical wisdom has held that the hip was something to be pinned together when elderly women fell, or to be replaced if and when the cartilage inside wore out during the senior years. For the rest of us, the ball-in-socket joint was viewed as a model of sturdy stability, of medical interest mostly when it was on the receiving end of trauma, such as when dislocated in a car accident or severely injured playing sports.

Dr. Kelly is one of an elite group of doctors specializing in hip dysfunction who realize that the hip is a lot more delicate than anyone has given it credit for. In the most common bad-news scenario, the hip joint is "impinged"—the ball of the femur doesn't have its full normal range of motion inside the socket—which then forces the pelvic joint in the center of the midsection to compensate with extra movement. The major abdominal muscle (the rectus abdominis) and the adductors that cross over the front of the pelvis get irritated by this movement and grow tight and

PROTECT YOUR LABRUM

When you get out of your car seat after a long drive, or your theater seat at the end of the movie, do your hips feels tight, achy, crampy? Perhaps the hip joint is "impinged" (suffers from an irritating, diminished range of motion), or a tear of the labrum could be part of the problem. Have an orthopedist check it out. In the meantime, back off of any strenuous activity at the first sign of hip pain. The labrum can be injured in accidents as well. Here's one common scenario: a car passenger rests his or her knees against the dashboard, and even a modest crash impact does the rest. When the hips are flexed at ninety degrees, the impact against the dashboard could tear the labrum.

painful. That's why Jane kept straining those core muscles, a syndrome that, as we mentioned before, doctors now call athletic pubalgia. In more serious cases such as hers, the orthopedist must repair the hip itself, cutting away some bone or the rim of the socket, to allow the joint to move more freely, and sewing up the hip's cartilage support, the labrum, which often gets torn by the pressures generated by that impinged hip.

It's a complex anatomy lesson, but it's important. The latest research suggests that this impingement/labral-tear combo is a time bomb inside the hip. It's a major cause for degeneration inside the joint, which over time often develops into osteoarthritis, and the need for hip replacement surgery.

Groin Pain: Psoas Impingement

Kathy, forty-two, is an executive with a New York media company who works hard and works out hard. She hikes, swims, cycles, you name it. But increasingly she's slowed down by groin pain, originally diagnosed as a simple groin pull. Because the pain is chronic and severe, Dr. Kelly suspects joint damage. He discovers that the source of the pain is actually muscular, the ropy iliopsoas, which runs from spine to thigh. It's now so tight, it's painfully pressing against the hip capsule along the way.

Dr. Kelly could surgically trim off some of the width of the psoas tendon, allowing for greater stretch and relieving the pressure on the hip. But by collaborating with Dr. DeStefano, he has the luxury of keeping the surgical option in reserve. Dr.

DeStefano does intensive manual work to break up the tension in the muscle, and after ten sessions Kathy is pain-free and back to hiking in Harriman State Park and hitting her weekly mileage marks on her bike.

As we've said quite a few times, our medical system tends to undervalue muscle damage in its eagerness to explain how pain and suffering is caused by structural problems inside the joints. Kathy's case is one example of a muscle disorder contributing to joint damage. Her case was resolved by working directly on the muscles. In more severe cases, when the tight iliopsoas tendon actually snaps against the hip capsule, surgery may be required to fix the situation.

Kathy's problem—a problem for a lot of us with demanding office jobs—is that she sits at her desk working long hours without taking regular walking and stretching breaks. Evolution hasn't designed us to be such good sitters. When the iliopsoas doesn't get a chance to do its primary job—flex the hip—it tightens up. Kathy is a regular exerciser, which is a good thing, but because she doesn't warm up before running, she irritated an already tight muscle. Even in less dramatic cases when the psoas isn't directly interfering with the hip, it still often refers pain from the hip to the groin area or the lower back.

Outer (Lateral) Hip Pain/Bursitis

The abductor muscles—the gluteus medius and minimus—have the nonstop job of stabilizing the pelvis. (They're the muscles that Sue strained with her clamshell exercises.) In middle age, playing two or three sets of tennis, formerly no big deal, can trigger pain in the outer-hip area. For the elderly, simply walking can bring on the pain. In both cases, the deconditioned abductors have fatigued, throwing off the position of the pelvis and the mechanics of moving, and maybe even irritating the protective bursa sac. (The major hip bursa lies outside the joint, near the protruding top part of the femur or thighbone called the greater trochanter, hence the name *trochanteric bursitis.*)

The standard treatment is rest and an anti-inflammatory injection if necessary. But once again, addressing the underlying muscle problem, either with manual therapy or surgery, depending on the severity of the damage, is changing the treatment landscape. Manual therapy to relieve muscle tightness along the iliotibial band, the long tendon that runs down the outside of the thigh, can relieve pressure on the bursa. (More about the iliotibial band in the next chapter.)

Leading hip surgeons have discovered that surgically repairing badly torn gluteus tendons is the key to solving what had been regarded as the toughest bursitis cases.

Joint/Orthopedic

Hip Impingement

You'll notice we put hip impingement in two categories: Muscle or Joint? and here in Joint/Orthopedic. In the case of Jane the marathoner, we had to tease out the muscle and joint issues to figure out that the compromised hip joint was at the root of her problems. But with a lot of the athletes Dr. Kelly sees—soccer, hockey, lacrosse players—there is no medical mystery. The friction in the impinged joint can tear the supporting cartilage and the labrum, increase instability and improper movement, and lead to pain. Surgery to reshape the hip socket and repair the labrum solves the problem, if it's caught in time. If not, bone grinding against bone inside the joint can lead to osteoarthritis and, ultimately, the need for joint replacement surgery.

Osteoarthritis

Marilyn is a fifty-year-old Manhattan corporate executive who came to Dr. Kelly with lower-back pain and limited mobility in both hips. She was overweight and

INFO

HIP RESURFACING (PARTIAL HIP REPLACEMENT)

Younger patients facing hip replacement may want to investigate an alternative to the standard surgery called hip resurfacing, or sometimes, a partial hip replacement. With the standard procedure, the femoral head (the ball that fits into the hip socket) is cut off and replaced with a metal prosthesis. With the newer procedure, which has been done in Europe for two decades but in this country only since 2006, the femoral head is shaved down and given a metal cup covering. More bone is preserved and the fit in the hip socket is closer, which may allow a greater range of motion and more active lifestyle. Both approaches have pros and cons. Research both options and discuss them with your orthopedist.

had no interest in exercise. Her goals were modest. All she wanted was to be able to walk without pain. Unfortunately, X-rays showed that her osteoarthritis was well advanced. She may have been genetically predisposed to the early onset of the disease, which had eaten away most of the cushioning cartilage in her hip joints. Or her weight and sedentary lifestyle may have been enough to send her over the edge. All the X-rays could tell Dr. Kelly was that the femoral heads, the balls in the ball-in-socket joint, were no longer round but flattened like a mushroom against the hip socket, bone on bone.

In Marilyn's case, Dr. Kelly appreciated that hip replacement surgery was inevitable, but that the timing was not yet right. Because the body will tolerate only a limited number of hip replacement operations in a lifetime, he wanted to buy as much time for Marilyn's God-given hips as he could. He referred her to Dr. DeStefano for regular treatment. Muscle therapy can relieve pain from the surrounding muscles, which contract in response to the distress signals sent out by the diseased joints. Marilyn can help herself by monitoring her diet (less weight means less pressure on the damaged joints) and engaging in low-impact exercise.

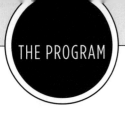

HIP

The major movements of the hip joint are flexion and extension (bend and straighten), adduction and abduction (move toward and away from the body), and external and internal rotation (twist the leg out and in). In other words, bringing the leg forward and back, bringing the legs together and apart, and twisting so the knee faces away from the body or toward it. The ball-and-socket joint makes all these variations possible, although the complex network of connective tissue also keeps the hip stable. Because so many muscles are attached to the hip, imbalances among them can affect the way the joint functions.

POSTERIOR THIGH

Purpose: To target and remove any restrictions and restore a full range of motion to the hamstring muscles and the whole kinetic chain of back muscles by manually releasing tight, short, and damaged muscles.

Starting out: Start by lying on your back with the both legs bent to ninety degrees at the hip and knee. Relax the muscles and grasp the treatment thigh with both hands with the fingers curved around the posterior leg. The pressure should be angled in and toward the hip. This large-muscle group can be divided into three zones: medial (inside), lateral (outside), and middle; and each long section can be divided into thirds or fourths, starting at the knee and moving toward the hip.

How to do it: Maintaining the angled pressure, lift the treatment leg off the floor, then straighten your knee, as far as is comfortable, without moving the thigh or causing pain. Hold for two seconds after the movement is completed. Repeat with your other leg. Complete three to four passes in each zone.

Troubleshooting: Don't press too hard too fast; let the hand "sink in." Avoid letting the skin slide under the hands by using angled pressure. The body should remain still and stable on the ground. Don't lower the thigh as the leg is straightened. It's better to start the movement with the bent leg lower, and straighten completely from there.

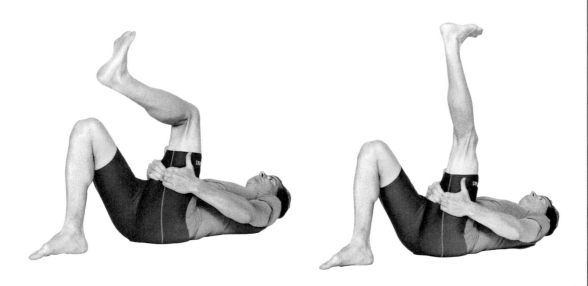

BUTTOCKS

Purpose: To target and remove any restrictions and restore a full range of motion to the gluteal region, including the piriformis and the external rotators, by manually releasing tight, short, and damaged muscles.

Starting out: Start by lying on your side with both legs extended. Grasp a tool (here we use a F.A.S.T. Stick™, but you can use a ball, etc.) and place it on the top hip in the muscle mass there. Stay off the bone at the side of the hip. The pressure should be angled in and up toward the back. This large-muscle group can be divided into three zones: medial, lateral, and middle; and each long section can be divided into thirds or fourths, starting at the base of the butt and moving up toward the back in each zone.

How to do it: Maintaining the angled pressure, bring the treatment knee up to the chest, as far as is comfortable, without causing pain. Hold for two seconds after the movement is completed. Repeat on the opposite side. Complete two to three passes in each zone.

Troubleshooting: Don't press too hard too fast; let the tool "sink in." Avoid letting the skin slide under the tool by using angled pressure. Keep the back and neck relaxed; don't strain and twist to hold the tool in place.

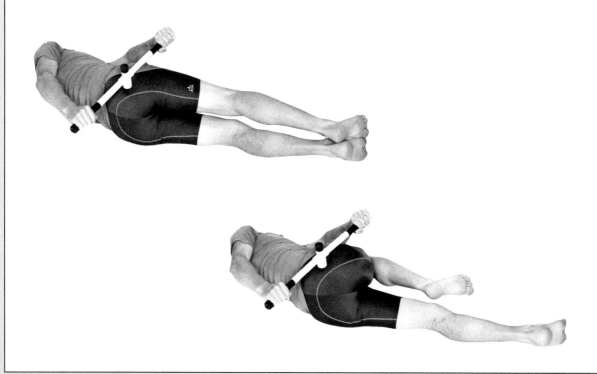

INNER THIGH

Purpose: To target and remove any restrictions and restore a full range of motion to the adductors by manually releasing tight, short, and damaged muscles.

Starting out: Start by lying on your back with one leg extended and the treatment leg bent up toward the chest. With pressure place the fingers of both hands on the inside of the thigh. (A F.A.S.T. Stick™ or other tool can also be used.) The pressure should be angled in and toward the hip. This large-muscle group can be divided into three zones: upper, middle, and lower; and each long section can be divided into thirds or fourths, starting at the base of the thigh and moving up toward the hip in each zone.

How to do it: Maintaining the angled pressure, allow the treatment leg to drop out to the side, as far as is comfortable, without causing pain or rolling to the side, then straighten the leg, also without causing pain or rolling. Hold for two seconds after the movement is completed. Bend the knee as you return to the starting position. Repeat with your other leg. Complete two to three passes in each zone.

Troubleshooting: Don't press too hard too fast; let your hand "sink in." Avoid letting the skin slide under your hands by using angled pressure. Keep your back and neck relaxed; don't strain and twist to hold your hands in place. Gently and slowly control the movement.

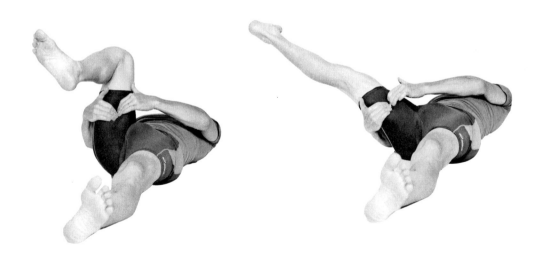

ANTERIOR THIGH

Purpose: To target and remove restrictions and restore a full range of motion to the quadriceps muscles, which can become contracted, notably the rectus femoris, which crosses the hip.

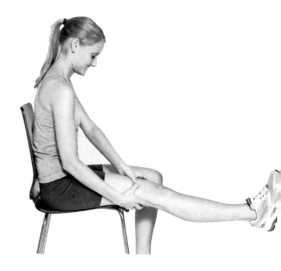

Starting out: Sit with one knee bent to ninety degrees, the foot flat on the floor. Extend the treatment leg out to the front. Place your hands on the quadriceps, grasping underneath the leg with the fingers and pushing the thumbs down and pulling up toward the body. An alternative grip for this large muscle is to grasp the quadriceps muscle as above, but place one thumb on top of the other, supporting and adding additional pressure to the first thumb. You can also use a tool. Because the quadriceps is a large muscle, the area must be broken down into three separate zones: inside, middle, and outside. Start working each zone about an inch and a half up from the knee and at three-inch intervals from there.

How to do it: With angular pressure applied to the quadriceps, bend the knee to ninety degrees, bringing the foot back past the other foot alongside the chair as far as is comfortable. Repeat with your other leg.

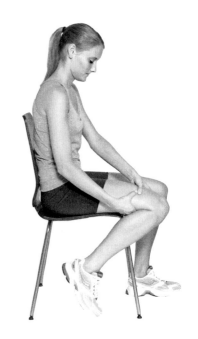

Troubleshooting: Do not apply too much pressure directly down into the muscle. Keep the pressure consistent and angled toward the hip. Do not slide the fingers over the skin and make sure to bend the knee as far as is possible without pain.

POSTERIOR THIGH

This stretch lengthens the hamstring, but the first part targets the attachment at the hip, gradually introducing more stretch as the knee extends. The straight leg stretches the whole muscle and both attachments at once and should only be done after the bent-knee stretch has warmed up the muscle. If the muscle is tight, this bent-knee stretch might be enough on its own.

Purpose: To warm up and lengthen the hamstrings. This can affect the whole posterior kinetic chain because of the significant connection with the lower-back musculature and because the hamstrings cross and affect the knee.

Starting out: Lie on your back with one leg outstretched and the treatment leg bent at ninety degrees. A rope should be looped around and across the ball of the treatment foot. The rope should be held firmly in both hands, with the knee in between the hands.

How to do it: Extend your leg from the knee as straight as is possible without moving the thigh or causing pain. At the end of the movement the rope can be used to gently bring the leg a little straighter, then stabilize the foot and hold the stretch in place for two seconds. Repeat with your other leg. The stretch should be repeated ten times.

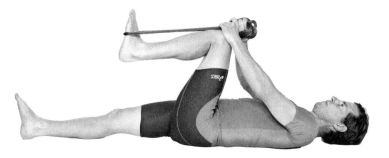

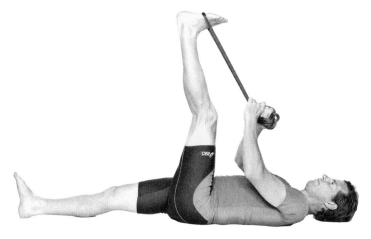

Advanced variation: This stretch starts out with the treatment leg straight and the other leg bent for stability. The rope is looped around your foot in the same way, although more rope is now necessary. Lift your leg as high as you comfortably can, while keeping it straight. Then you can use the rope to pull gently—only if necessary—to deepen the stretch, though the rope should mainly help to stabilize and hold the stretch for two seconds. Repeat with your other leg. Repeat ten times. Do this stretch after the bent-knee stretch has been completed.

Troubleshooting: Your body should remain still and stable on the ground. Your leg should remain in a straight line and not drop off to the side. Nothing is gained by overstretching, so respect the limits of the hamstring and only straighten to the point of a *gentle stretch.* The rope is not a crank for the leg—use it for stabilization, not a tug-of-war with your hamstring. Only apply a gentle tension with the rope at the end of the movement, not throughout.

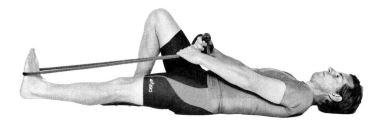

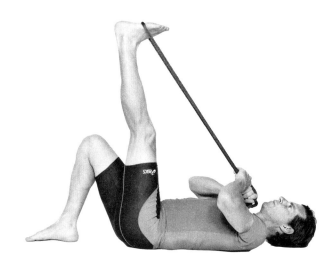

BUTTOCKS

Purpose: To warm up and lengthen the piriformis, the gluteus muscles, and the muscles of external rotation.

Starting out: Lie on your back with one leg bent at ninety degrees at the hip and at the knee. The treatment leg should be crossed over the other leg with the ankle resting on the knee.

How to do it: Grasp the far leg with both hands at the midthigh and pull both legs toward the chest. Switch leg positions and repeat. The stretch should be held for two seconds and repeated ten times.

Troubleshooting: Allow your back and head to rest flat on the ground. Only pull the legs far enough to feel a gentle stretch. Stop immediately if there is uncomfortable pressure or pain in the lower back, knee, or hip joint.

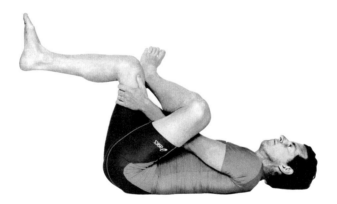

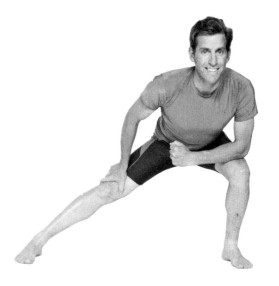

INNER THIGH

Purpose: To warm up and lengthen the adductors.

Starting out: Stand with a wide stance (wider than shoulders' width, but only as wide as is comfortable). With an upright posture and a flat back, bend your knees.

How to do it: Shift your weight to one side, touching your hand or forearm to the leg for two seconds. Contracting the abdominals and back muscles, shift to the other side, touching down for two seconds. Repeat ten times to each side in a controlled, rhythmic motion.

Troubleshooting: Don't use momentum; keep the motion slow and controlled. Do not lean too far forward or put too much body weight on the thigh. Keep your weight evenly distributed over your feet. Stop immediately if there is uncomfortable pressure in the knee or hip joint.

SELF-TREATMENT · STRETCHES · EXERCISES ·

ANTERIOR THIGH

Purpose: To warm up and lengthen the quadriceps.

Starting out: Start out lying on your side with both knees pulled to your chest. The bottom leg should be held at the knee, and the top, treatment leg should be held at the ankle.

How to do it: Bring the treatment leg back, foot first, so that your heel is closer to your glutes. The stretch should be felt on the front of the thigh and should be held for two seconds only. Switch sides and repeat with your other leg. Repeat ten times.

Troubleshooting: Be sure to keep the bottom leg stable and pulled into the chest. If the ankle of the treatment leg can't be comfortably grasped and moved, a rope can be used. Stop immediately if there is uncomfortable pressure in the knee or hip joint.

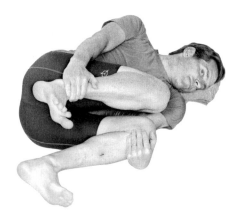
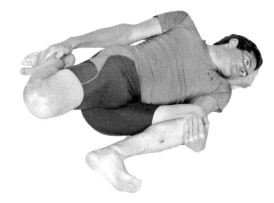

POSTERIOR THIGH

SUPERMAN KICKS

Purpose: To strengthen the muscles of the hamstrings, the glutes, and the lower back, as well as the core and posterior kinetic chain in general. This contributes to posture and balance, as well as general spine health. This also serves to warm up the muscles and prevent strain on other structures.

Starting: Lie facedown with your legs together and extended. Your arms should be crossed under your head.

How to do it: Slowly flex the knee, bringing the heel closer to the buttocks, as far as is comfortable and without pain. In a controlled manner, return the leg to the full extension of the starting position. Repeat with your other leg. Do two to three sets of ten to fifteen repetitions, held for no more than two seconds each.

Advanced variation: When the knee is flexed, push your heel up toward the ceiling, engaging the glutes. Relax your upper body; don't arch the back. Keep lifting your leg at the end, increasing the load on the glutes and making this a combination glute/hamstring move.

Troubleshooting: Do not move too quickly or pause at the top and the bottom of the exercise: keep the movement fluid and controlled. Do not use an ankle weight that is too heavy to keep proper form and pace. Keep the body relaxed—do not arch the back or the neck or recruit other muscles to help.

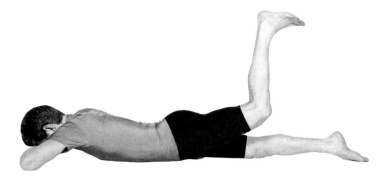

BUTTOCKS

SUPERMAN LEG RAISES

Purpose: To strengthen the muscles of the lower back, the glutes, and the hamstrings, as well as the core and posterior kinetic chain in general. This contributes to posture and balance, as well as general spine health. This will also warm up the muscles and help prevent strain on other structures of the upper body.

Starting out: Lie facedown with your legs together and extended. Your arms should be crossed under your head.

How to do it: Squeeze your glutes and legs and stabilize by contracting your abdominals and shoulder blades. One at a time, lift one straightened leg, then the other. Hold each for a count of two. Do ten repetitions.

Advanced variation: Ankle weights can be used to make the exercise more challenging. Alternately, both legs can be lifted at the same time (support the lower back by contracting the abdominals).

Troubleshooting: Do not release the stabilizing contraction of the lower and middle body. Keep your eyes looking at the floor and your head relaxed. Remember to breathe and don't clench your teeth. Keep the toe pointed and move the leg as one unit from the hip. Don't worry about how high you can lift the leg—think about how long you can stretch it while lifting.

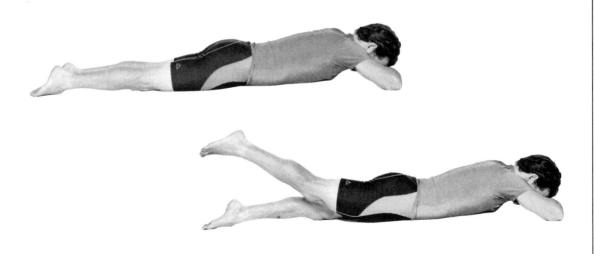

INNER THIGH

BODY-WEIGHT SQUAT

Purpose: To strengthen the adductors, although a body-weight squat also works the quadriceps, hamstrings, glutes, back, and stabilizing muscles of the core and joints.

Starting out: Stand with your feet wider than shoulders' width apart, feet parallel, and weight distributed evenly over your heels and toes.

How to do it: Hold your hands out in front of you, on your hips, or behind your head. Keeping a straight back, bend your knees, lowering the buttocks down toward the floor until the hip reaches knee level, or as far as is possible with good form and no pain. Keep your weight distributed evenly over your feet. Contract your glutes, abdominals, and quadriceps, and squeeze your legs together to bring the body back to the starting position. Contracting the adductors will prevent your knees from splaying out. Do ten repetitions, held for no more than two seconds each.

Troubleshooting: The depth of the squat should be challenging but should not disrupt good form or timely set completion. Keep your eyes looking forward, your back straight, and your head relaxed. Remember to breathe and don't clench your teeth. Don't lock your knees at the top or let them splay in or out during the movement. Keep your weight evenly distributed across the feet—don't rock onto your toes or heels—and don't lean forward. If there is a sharp pain in the groin or the knees, stop and seek medical counsel.

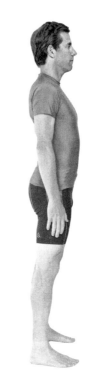

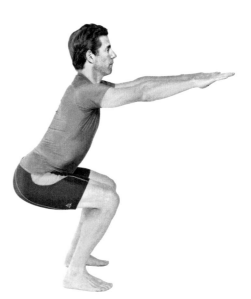

SELF-TREATMENT • STRETCHES • EXERCISES •

ANTERIOR THIGH

SQUAT WITH KETTLE BELL

Purpose: To strengthen the quadriceps, although a front squat also works the hamstrings, glutes, back, and stabilizing muscles of the core and the body as they pertain to balance and safe back movement.

Starting out: Stand with your feet wider than shoulders' width apart, feet turned slightly out. Hold a kettle bell with both hands, letting it hang in front of the hips. If a kettle bell is not available, any weight (dumbbell, can of soup) can be used as long as it is firmly held.

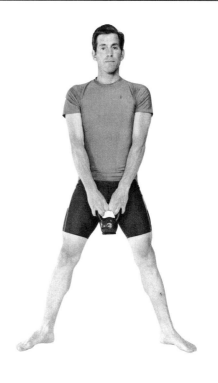

How to do it: Keeping a straight back, bend your knees, lowering the weight toward the floor until your hips reach knee level, or as far as is possible with good form and no pain. Contract the glutes, abdominals, quadriceps, and adductors to bring the body back to the starting position. Do ten repetitions, held for no more than two seconds each.

Troubleshooting: The weight should be challenging but should not disrupt good form or timely set completion. Keep your eyes looking forward, your back straight, and your head relaxed. Remember to breathe and don't clench your teeth. Don't lock your knees at the top or let them splay in or out during the movement. Keep your weight evenly distributed across your feet—don't rock onto your toes or heels— and don't lean forward. If a pain occurs in the groin or the knees, stop and seek medical counsel.

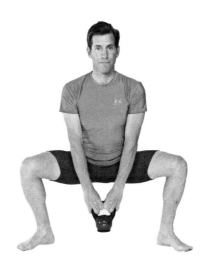

FULL BODY/CORE

A. SINGLE-LEG TOE TOUCH

See page 167.

B. KETTLE BELL SWING

See page 168.

THE KNEE

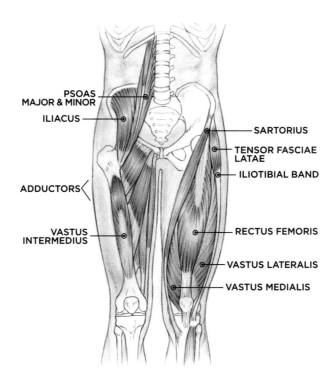

PSOAS MAJOR & MINOR

ILIACUS

SARTORIUS

TENSOR FASCIAE LATAE

ILIOTIBIAL BAND

ADDUCTORS

VASTUS INTERMEDIUS

RECTUS FEMORIS

VASTUS LATERALIS

VASTUS MEDIALIS

INTRODUCING THE KNEE

The knee, along with the ankle, is probably the most injured joint in the body. Tearing the anterior cruciate ligament (ACL) is, unfortunately, a common injury in turning/twisting sports such as skiing and soccer. Tearing the meniscus cartilage is an all too common occurence for ex-jock and couch potato alike. Trouble can arrive with a sudden pop and the onset of pain and swelling, but it may have been

IMMEDIATE TREATMENT/
WHEN TO SEE A DOCTOR

Sudden pain followed by swelling and difficulty straightening the knee or walking all suggest a serious tendon or ligament tear. Get medical attention. Likewise, if the knee "catches" or locks. As with any joint problem, check for any signs of infection—redness, heat or fever, and pain not connected to changes in activity. If there are any, see a doctor immediately. When the dire possibilities have been ruled out, you can assume you've got some kind of soft-tissue damage, usually a strain or sprain. The normal rules of RICE apply: Rest (keep weight off the area); Ice it; keep inflammation down with Compression (a compression bandage); and Elevation (bring the affected area above the level of your heart). It's your call whether to seek out a doctor or therapist right away, but if you still can't put weight on your leg after one week, it's time.

brewing from years or decades of overuse, poor sports form, or silently deteriorating connective tissue.

The machinery inside the knee joint gets so much attention that it might be tempting to assume that the muscles around the joint play a lesser role. But that's not the case. As discussed, the muscles soak up impact shock when the leg strikes the ground, helping the joint to resist injury. When injury does occur—let's say the ACL tears—we can't just focus on the joint damage to the exclusion of the other two elements of that interconnected system: bone and muscle. Unless we work on relaxing and strengthening the quadriceps and hamstring muscles, ideally before and definitely after joint surgery, that knee may not heal as well and may still have problems after surgery.

The way the knee is put together gives you an idea of its strength and its weakness. It's basically two large bones, the femur (thigh) and the tibia (lower leg), that form a hinge that is lashed together by a latticework of connective tissue. The third bone, the patella or kneecap, is suspended in a tendinous sheath in front of the joint, moving up and down in a groove in the femur. The smaller lower-leg bone, the fibula, creates its own joint with the tibia, providing crucial support for the knee.

COMMON PROBLEMS AND CULPRITS

The four thigh muscles, the quadriceps, are the brutes of the front-of-the-knee region. They bring the lower leg forward by straightening the knee joint. The longest of the quads, the rectus femoris, also flexes the hip, the only one of the four muscles that crosses both joints. Running beside the rectus femoris are the vastus lateralis on the out-side, and the vastus medialis on the inside, with the vastus intermedius beneath. Quad muscles occasionally tear from extreme exertion; more typically they overpower one of the others. If a stronger vastus lateralis overpowers a vastus medialis, the result can be a mistracking kneecap and painful "runner's knee."

The three major muscles behind the knee, the hamstrings, counter the quads. The hamstrings pull the lower leg back by flexing the knee joint and they extend the hip. They are prone to strain, although chronic hamstring pulls are fairly rare outside the world of high-level sports. A small muscle behind the knee, the popliteus, helps flex and stabilize the joint. Although mainstream medicine doesn't pay too much attention to the popliteus, many manual therapists find that it is often strained in runners and have had good success treating it manually.

The iliotibial (IT) band (functionally the long tendon of a short hip muscle, the ten-sor fasciae latae, and the gluteus maximus) runs down the outside of the leg, from the crest of the pelvis to the top of the tibia. It acts largely as a brace, keeping both the femur in place on the tibia and stabilizing the extended knee. Overuse, typically from running, can irritate the IT band and cause nagging pain along the outer side of the leg, especially at the knee and the hip.

The joint is sturdy enough to handle the tremendous forces generated by two of the strongest muscle groups in the body, the quadriceps and the hamstrings. At the same time, it's vulnerable. It doesn't have a solid bony covering like the hip or the elbow so the ligaments that hold the joint in place are an easy target in a collision.

The knee is not a simple hinge like the elbow. It bends and straightens, but it also slightly rotates. Its rounded ends roll over the flat top surface of the tibia, which allows for more mobility. You can plant your foot and cut—shift direction—as you run. What makes this extra movement of the bones possible are the menisci, two crescent-shaped pieces of fibrocartilage in between the femur and the tibia that act as shock absorbers. It's a wonderful system, until it takes a direct hit or the pieces begin to wear out.

WHAT GOES WRONG, AND HOW TO FIX IT

Mostly Muscular

Front-of-Knee Pain: Patellofemoral Pain Syndrome or "Runner's Knee"
Chris, then a twenty-year-old triathlete, was confiding to the manager of his local New Jersey bike shop that he was leaving the sport because he couldn't take the knee pain anymore. His training runs irritated the front of his knee, generating a dull, nonspecific ache that a lot of runners are familiar with—patellofemoral pain syndrome or "runner's knee." None of the doctors or therapists he'd seen had been of any help. Dr. DeStefano, a recreational triathlete, overheard him in the store and offered to help. Chris's kneecap, it turned out, was not tracking properly. The quadriceps muscle that pulls the kneecap to the inside, the vastus medialis, was being overwhelmed by the vastus lateralis, which pulls to the outside. As a consequence, Chris's kneecap was painfully rubbing against the groove in the femur in which it rides. After three weeks of manual work to lessen tightness in all four of the quad muscles and then physical therapy to strengthen the vastus medialis in particular, the problem was resolved. Chris, now thirty-four, competes as a professional triathlete.

The quadriceps are almost always at the root of front-of-

SELF-DEFENSE

PROTECT YOUR KNEES

Avoid prolonged squatting, for instance, when doing housework or gardening.

Avoid heels that are over one inch as much as possible.

Don't prop your feet up on a table without some support under your knees.

Don't sit with one leg tucked underneath you or sit on the floor with your legs to the side.

Jog conservatively. Unless you're in serious training, try not to run more than every other day (cross-train on the off-days) and try to stick to softer running surfaces.

the-knee problems. The simplest injury is a quad strain—the muscle fires too hard or too rapidly, and swelling or bruising results. Athletes in high-impact sports such as basketball or high jumping can generate so much muscular force that the tissues around the tendon connecting the quads to the kneecap become inflamed, causing patellar tendonosis or "jumper's knee." But the problem that derailed Chris, and derails countless joggers, is patellofemoral pain. Sometimes there's a mild puffiness around the kneecap, and sometimes not, but the constant ache can make the knee feel like a rusty hinge.

The term *patellofemoral pain* tells us where the problem is located but doesn't give us any clue as to what's causing it. There are many different muscle imbalances and joint abnormalities that can add up to a mistracking kneecap.

Women tend to have greater Q angles, which contribute to a running gait that can pull the kneecap to the outside. (Statistics show that females have a greater incidence of front-of-the-knee pain than males.) A kneecap that rides unusually high can also create problems. Fortunately, whatever the cause, the prescription is almost always the same, muscle treatment—and self-treatment—then strength work.

Outside (Lateral) Knee Pain: Iliotibial Band Pain Syndrome

Runners have another familiar enemy, a tight IT band. This dense, fibrous band of tissue runs down the outside of the hip and thigh to the top of the tibia. Under ordinary circumstances, the IT band provides some extra stability for the knee (which can always use it). But when the IT band tightens up from overuse, it can rub against the bony outer edge of the knee, generating anything from a dull ache to a sharp, stabbing pain. The mechanics here appear to be straightforward, but if we work our way back up the "kinetic chain" to find the source of the problem, we may discover other explanations for IT band irritation. For instance, the left side of the patient's lumbar spine may be tight, causing a decrease in left spinal rotation and forcing an overrotation to the right. This causes the right leg to strike the ground with extra force, irritating the IT band. The manual therapist then works on the lower-back muscles as well as the knee muscles to fix the problem.

Often what gets labeled as IT band pain syndrome is just the muscles on that side of the leg causing pain and dysfunction. True IT band pain syndrome causes locking of the knee and severe pain on the outside of the knee.

Muscle or Joint?

Meniscus Tear

In her late fifties, Sister Carol Zinn serves as a high-powered liaison between the Catholic Church and the United Nations. One day, she missed a step walking down some stairs and landed hard on her right foot. Without time to contract her leg muscles, the impact shock traveled straight to her knee joint. The jolt was only mildly painful, but over the next few hours the joint became swollen. She was left with a constant dull ache and a sharp pain when she flexed her knee. Dr. DeStefano saw her a few days later and began manually working on all the major muscles that support the knee, but progress was slow. He sent Sister Carol to Dr. Kelly, who found a torn meniscus on an MRI, but nevertheless decided the damage didn't warrant surgery. He gave her a corticosteroid injection, which calmed the area down and allowed her to make an important overseas trip. For the two years since then, Dr. DeStefano has successfully kept her pain at bay with regular manual treatment, and Sister Carol continues to travel constantly.

In Sister Carol's case, her damaged meniscus was without a doubt the source of the problem. The question was whether the meniscus needed to be surgically removed or whether her condition could be managed by concentrating on the traumatized muscles.

We like to say that the MRI has its pros and cons. Having such an accurate picture of what's going on inside the joint can help us make more accurate diagnoses, but it can also reveal incidental findings that are not the cause of the pain. The meniscus is a case in point. Unlike an X-ray, an MRI will reveal a tear in the meniscus, but it can't always tell us whether the tear happened last week or last decade. In Sister Carol's case, she may have torn the cartilage by landing hard on that step, or an old tear might have left the knee more susceptible to the force of the impact.

In any event, the injury shut down the surrounding muscles. Inflammation triggered muscle pain and a buildup of fluid around the joint. The most conservative step was to work on those muscles, first with manual therapy to speed up healing, then with physical therapy to make them strong enough to compensate for the lack of a healthy, stabilizing meniscus. The goal isn't a perfect knee, just one that functions as well as it possibly can. In Sister Carol's case, a single injection of an anti-inflammatory corticosteroid worked wonders. But lacking the support of a healthy meniscus, her knee is still prone to irritation and tightness; she sees Dr. DeStefano for treatment every couple of weeks.

Sometimes it is a fresh meniscus tear that is the source of difficulty. Typically, a piece of the torn cartilage gets trapped between the femur and the tibia, causing pain or the joint to "catch" or "lock." Here, surgery is the likely option, but only to remove the troublemaking piece of tissue. Again, if older people, with the help of therapy and anti-inflammatories, can comfortably get by without meniscus surgery, they probably should. There's a particular reason for this. All too often, the meniscus tear is the consequence of wear-and-tear deterioration affecting all the cartilage in the knee. The missed step or the awkward twist is just the proverbial straw that broke the camel's back. If the articular cartilage that allows the femur and the tibia to move smoothly against each other is in similarly bad shape, then knee replacement surgery looms on the horizon. There's little point to subjecting the patient to a meniscus surgery if the whole knee will shortly be replaced.

Young people are looking at a different scenario. If they tear a meniscus, it's most likely the result of trauma. If

INFO

KNEE STATS

According to the latest statistics, between the ages of twenty-five and seventy-five, your chance of having disabling knee pain or injury is about 50 percent. About one in five Americans over age sixty has chronic knee pain, compared to one in seven for chronic hip pain.

the tear is small enough, the pain and swelling may subside so quickly the damage never gets diagnosed (perhaps to show up on an MRI twenty years later). For a more serious injury, the location of the tear may determine the treatment. When discussing surgery, there really isn't such a thing as an "unnecessary surgery." Orthopedics repair damaged structures because they are damaged. The question is whether that structural damage is causing the patient's symptoms. As with a lot of orthopedic procedures, the question isn't whether meniscus surgery is good or bad, but good or bad for whom, and under what conditions: Sister Carol or a twenty-year-old point guard?

Joint/Orthopedic

ACL (and Other Ligament) Tears

In skiing, all it takes to tear your ACL is landing off-balance after going over a mogul. Dr. DeStefano treated a well-known U.S. skier who had suffered a total body blow after flying off a downhill course at full speed. Luckily, her most serious injury was a torn ACL. Well into the 1980s, the standard treatment would have been to rush her into surgery, then put her knee in a hard cast, inadvertently ensuring that the traumatized muscles would completely atrophy and the knee joint would freeze shut with scar tissue that would have to be painfully broken up in physical therapy. Now, we wait several weeks before surgery. We let the inflammation subside and we build up the muscle strength and the joint's range of motion. Dr. DeStefano had such good results manually working on the skier's supporting knee muscles (mostly the quads and the hamstrings), she felt like she didn't need the ACL surgery after all. When her ACL was tested, the tibia still slid out from under the femur; strong muscles might hold her knee together for everyday life, but not for barreling down a ski run at seventy miles per hour. But all the muscle work had set her up beautifully for the surgery, the flexible cast, and the rehab that followed. She returned to competition, where she added several medals to her collection before she retired.

The two cruciate ligaments (the anterior cruciate ligament, or ACL, and the posterior cruciate ligament, or PCL) cross each other inside the knee joint, hence the name *cruciate,* which means "cross." They keep the tibia and femur stable by preventing forward or backward movement of the tibia under the femur. The two collateral ligaments (the lateral collateral ligament, or LCL, and the medial collateral ligament, or MCL) keep the two leg bones from sliding side to side. A single collision or violent motion can injure one or any combination of them.

Depending on which way the knee moves after it's hit, the ligaments will tear in a predictable sequence, and these multiple ligament injuries are usually the most challenging to treat. But the ACL is the most frequently injured and is the star ligament that receives the most attention in the sports medicine and media worlds. Injure it and you may hear a pop, then feel the pain and endure the swelling.

The decision to surgically reconstruct the ACL is not automatic. For older people whose idea of the sporting life is a nice, brisk walk, a knee with a torn ACL and compromised stability may be good enough, especially if they commit to therapy to relax and strengthen the joint muscles. Unlike with meniscus tears, age isn't always an overriding factor in the decision to operate. If your torn ACL means you can't walk across the street without your knee buckling, you're a surgical candidate even if you do carry an AARP card. However, if joint replacement surgery is in your near future, having two major knee

PROTECT YOUR ACL

Wear well-fitted athletic shoes. If you have a bow-legged or knock-kneed gait that results from your foot structure, consider orthotic inserts for your shoes.

Be in top physical condition for your sport; make sure the leg muscles are strong and balanced.

Work with a competent coach on proper sports form and technique.

surgeries within a few years of each other is probably not a good idea. Wearing a brace can be a workable stopgap solution for an unstable knee.

For a younger person, especially someone active in sports, ACL surgery is pretty much a slam-dunk decision. Pivoting and jumping without the ligament is just an invitation to further injury and the fast track to osteoarthritis. (Ligaments outside the joint capsule do have the capacity to heal themselves, but there will likely be some permanent loss of strength and support.) Fortunately, ACL reconstruction is one of the great success stories of modern orthopedics—

ACL RECONSTRUCTION

INFO

Most ACL reconstructions are done as "minimally invasive" surgery, with an arthroscope. A small fiber-optic camera is inserted into the joint so the procedure, performed with delicate instruments, can be monitored on a video screen. The surgeon harvests a new piece of replacement connective tissue from the patella or hamstring tendon and screws it into place using holes drilled into the femur and tibia. Sometimes, donor tissue from a cadaver is used instead.

positive outcomes are in the mid-90 percent range. This success story owes much to improvements in surgical technique (see the "ACL Reconsruction" box above), and also to orthopedists paying closer attention to the muscles that ultimately have to be able to drive the joint and the leg. As the story of the skier shows, treating and strengthening the muscles before and after surgery can greatly reduce the recovery and rehabilitation time. And your knee will probably function better, sooner.

In the last few years, the sports medicine world has begun to appreciate the connection between the bone structure of the knee and the ACL tear. The latest research shows that women injure their ACLs at over twice the rate of men. In sports such as soccer, volleyball, and basketball, where both sexes play according to similar rules, the female rate of ACL injury may be as much as five times as high. As we said earlier, women generally have a larger Q angle—wider hips create a steeper line from the hip to the knee—which is likely one factor that explains the difference between injury rates. Women's weight also falls more on the inside of the knee, which can overstress the ACL. A running gait where the knees pull toward the midline is a sign of a large Q angle and a potential problem (see the Self-Defense box on page 205).

Osteoarthritis

Several years ago, we treated a top amateur marathoner and triathlete in his late thirties. Let's call him Sam. We discovered that a hip-muscle imbalance was causing his knee muscles to overcontract. As a consequence, the femur and the tibia were twisting against each other, progressively shearing away the protective articular cartilage. In addition, some osteoarthritis had developed. We told Sam he had only a few good options: a sustained course of manual therapy to resolve the hip problem, physical therapy for the knee injury, and a cut back on the running. A hard-charging Manhattan business executive, Sam sought a second opinion that suited him better: several rounds of cortisone injections to quiet the inflammation, no lifestyle change required. Eventually, Sam underwent joint replacement surgery to replace his osteoarthritis-ridden right knee. But being hardheaded isn't all bad. He's since switched to cycling and is now one of the top amateur cyclists in his area.

Doctors sometimes like to use the analogy of a tire when they're trying to get the attention of patients whose knees have begun to show signs of osteoarthritis: "You have this much tread left. Do you want to keep jogging and use it up in six months to a year, or do you want to try to keep your knees for longer?" What patients sometimes fail to appreciate is that while it may have taken twenty or thirty

OSTEOARTHRITIS

There is no known cure for arthritis; we manage it. Weight control is essential. In climbing stairs, an extra 50 pounds translates to 150 to 200 pounds of extra pressure on your knees. High-impact exercise such as running is out; low-impact exercise such as swimming or cycling or the elliptical-trainer machine is in. Rhythmic movement that doesn't jar the joints and stimulates the production of lubricating synovial fluid can only help. Recent research shows that building muscle strength with weight training can help—start slowly and gradually increase the intensity of the exercise. Pain can be managed with anti-inflammatory drugs and, if necessary, occasional corticosteroid injections. Advances in manual medicine suggest that by releasing tightness in the surrounding muscles, manual therapy may lessen the pressure on the joint capsule, reducing the friction of bone moving against bone and slowing the progression of the disease. The goal may be to hold off severe, disabling arthritis indefinitely or to buy time so that if a patient anticipates knee replacement down the line, only one surgery is necessary.

INFO

THE "MINI-KNEE" AND TIBIAL OSTEOTOMY

If arthritis is present in only part of your knee joint, you could be a candidate for a partial or "unicompartmental" knee replacement, nicknamed the mini-knee, which leaves the healthy portion of the joint untouched. Younger patients whose arthritis is contained are good candidates for a procedure called a tibial osteotomy where a wedge of the shinbone is removed from the healthy side of the knee so that pressure is directed away from the diseased, arthritic portion. The goal of both procedures is to buy time, as much as a decade, before replacing the whole knee, reducing the chance of needing more than one total replacement in a lifetime.

years of pounding the pavement to trigger the disease, once osteoarthritis has set in, the knee can go from sore but functional to almost useless in months.

Our osteoarthritis patients tend to fall into two camps. They're like Sam, who aggravates the problem in the pursuit of competition, fitness, and feel-good endorphins. Or they're older, often in their sixties or seventies, and unaware that they're subjecting the knee to unusual stress. Influenced by genetics or by knee injuries sustained earlier in life, their articular cartilage silently wears away until one day knee pain announces itself, or their altered biomechanics may cause a meniscal tear.

Focal Chondral Injury

Not all damage to the knee's articular cartilage is from wear and tear. Blows to the knee, typically in sports, can damage a segment of cartilage right down to the bone. If you're under forty, and the health of the rest of your cartilage is good, you should be able to take advantage of one of a growing number of surgical procedures that either replaces the injured area with a cartilage graft or encourages new cartilage to grow. If the "focal defect" isn't fixed, it may set in motion the downward slide to "global" osteoarthritis.

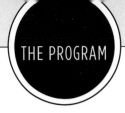

KNEE

The knee has two movements that concern us here: flexion and extension (bend and straighten). While the joint also allows for some medial and lateral rotation, there is certainly not enough movement to protect it from the torquing forces put on it in life and sports, which can cause discomfort and injury. The knee muscles' main functions are to propel the body and to cushion impact, and the best way for you to assist the joint is to maintain the balance and strength of those supporting muscles.

ANTERIOR THIGH

See page 186.

LATERAL THIGH

Purpose: To self-treat the iliotibial band (ITB). This is important for movement and stabilization of the knee. The IT band can adhere to the vastus lateralis, causing dysfunction in that muscle and causing friction at the IT band's attachment at the knee.

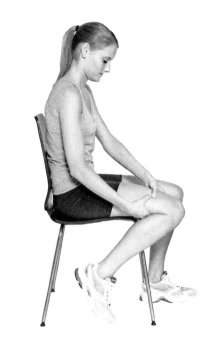

Starting out: Sit with both feet on the floor and the treatment leg bent to forty-five degrees. Using both hands, apply pressure down onto the IT band and angle the pressure either up toward the body or down toward the knee. There is one zone, running along the lateral leg from the knee to the hip. Start working about three inches up from the knee and at three-inch intervals from there.

How to do it: Maintaining the angled pressure, extend your leg. A F.A.S.T. Stick™ or other tool can also be used to apply pressure. Repeat with your other leg.

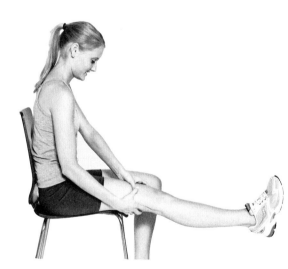

Troubleshooting: This self-treatment has to be slow without too much pressure as the tendon can become irritated. Gentle pressure should help relieve tightness, which can occur between the tendon and the underlying muscles.

POSTERIOR THIGH

See page 183.

See also self-treatment for the tibialis anterior on page 223.

ANTERIOR THIGH

See page 191.

LATERAL THIGH
(See illustrations on page 191.)

Purpose: To warm up and lengthen the IT band and the structures around it. This is the same as the quadriceps stretch with a variation.

Starting out: Start out lying on your side with both knees pulled to the chest. Your bottom leg should be held at the knee, and the top, treatment leg should be held at the ankle.

How to do it: Bring the treatment leg back, foot first so that the heel is closer to the glutes. Drop the leg down, allowing it to sink as far to the floor as is comfortable. Switch sides and repeat with your other leg. This should be held for two seconds only. Repeat ten times.

Troubleshooting: Be sure to keep your bottom leg stable and pulled to the chest. If the ankle of the treatment leg can't be comfortably grasped and moved, use a rope or band. Stop immediately if there is uncomfortable pressure in the knee or hip joint.

POSTERIOR THIGH

See page 187.

ANTERIOR THIGH

See page 195.

LATERAL THIGH

The IT band is a tendon, not a muscle. Connective tissue can be treated and stretched, but it cannot be strengthened like a muscle. Exercises that generally contribute to IT band strength appear in the hip-exercises section (pages 193–196).

POSTERIOR THIGH

See page 192.

FULL BODY/CORE

A. SINGLE-LEG TOE TOUCH

See page 167.

B. KETTLE BELL SWING

See page 168.

C. BODY-WEIGHT SQUAT

See page 194.

D. SQUAT WITH KETTLE BELL

See page 195.

THE ANKLE AND THE FOOT

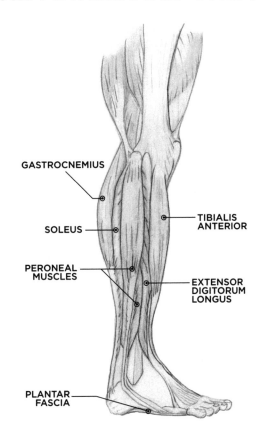

GASTROCNEMIUS

SOLEUS

PERONEAL
MUSCLES

TIBIALIS
ANTERIOR

EXTENSOR
DIGITORUM
LONGUS

PLANTAR
FASCIA

INTRODUCING THE ANKLE AND THE FOOT

The last hot spot, the ankle and the foot, is of course where your body makes contact with the ground, roughly five thousand to ten thousand times a day. That's an amazing amount of pounding. You want that foot plant to be stable and secure,

SPORTS PODIATRIST DAN GELLER

Health professionals are going to see what they're trained to see. Some orthopedists may not be interested in a case unless there's a surgical issue. The podiatrist is going to say, "You're pronating, that's the root of all evil." But as an athlete, I know there's not just one fix. Orthotics can be a great adjunct, but they can be overprescribed or wrongly prescribed—as when the material or the design doesn't fit the foot in question. And just because someone is injured, doesn't mean they need an orthotic. Maybe they need to replace their shoes, stop training so hard, and stay off the hills for a while. As a clinician, you have to get out of the mind-set of wanting to be the hero by fixing them. You're really doing the right thing when you put the patient in the right hands. For instance, some of my patients have done really well working on muscular issues with Dr. DeStefano.

especially if you're active in sports. If this first link in the kinetic chain is weak—if something is off about the way bones, joints, and muscles work together to move you around—the impact that travels up through the foot and the ankle will likely result in some kind of lower-extremity injury. It could be an overuse injury. When the connective tissue that forms the major arch in the foot gets inflamed, it's called plantar fasciitis. When the outer shinbone tissue gets irritated, it's medial tibial stress syndrome, or shin splints. Or it could be a trauma. You step in a pothole and turn your ankle, and the ligaments and muscles aren't resilient enough to prevent an ankle sprain, the single most common musculoskeletal injury. Chicago Bulls all-time great Michael Jordan was famous for avoiding the foot and leg injuries that often sideline pro basketball players. Every day he would religiously do stretching and strengthening exercises similar to the ones you'll find at the end of this chapter.

The ankle is a pretty simple design. Technically speaking, it's a mortise joint, *mortise* being a carpentry term for the space that something else fits into. The two bones of the lower leg, the tibia and the fibula, create a squarish space that houses the ankle bone or talus. The foot, by contrast, is an incredibly complex collection of 26 bones (almost one-fourth of the body's total), 33 joints, 107 ligaments, and more than 7,000 nerve endings. Together, they make an effective combo.

As your foot makes contact with the ground, the ankle flexes, then the calf muscles contract and push your weight onto the balls of the foot and the toes, propelling you forward. The foot's bones, ligaments, and muscles support the entire weight of your body, or up to eight times your body weight if you're running. What makes this possible is the curved architecture of the foot—three arches that absorb shock by flattening on impact, then springing back to their original shape during push off. The ankle's side-to-side flexibility allows the foot to find a stable platform as it moves through uneven terrain. Ligaments on both the inside and the outside of the ankle are the key structural element that holds the ankle bones in place as you suddenly change direction when running. If the foot turns too far to either side (usually twisting to the outside in a stumble), the all-too-common ankle sprain is the result.

As you've seen in our discussion of the other hot spots, musculoskeletal problems are conventionally divided up between orthopedists, who concentrate on structural damage, and physical and muscle therapists, who work on muscles. (This entire book is an argument against this either/or thinking, since most injuries are a specific mix of both muscular and structural elements.) The foot/ankle hot zone is sufficiently complicated to support a third group of health professionals, the podiatrists, who zero in on the biomechanics of the foot, typically problems with the arches. The distinctive tool in their toolbox is the prescription arch support, or

RED
FLAG

IMMEDIATE TREATMENT/
WHEN TO SEE A DOCTOR

It's often hard to tell whether you've sprained or broken the ankle. But if you can't put weight on it, it's likely either a severe sprain or a fracture. Get medical treatment. As with any joint problem, check for any signs of infection—redness, heat or fever, and pain not connected to changes in activity. If there are any, see a doctor immediately. When the dire possibilities have been ruled out, you can assume you've got some kind of less serious soft-tissue damage, a ligament sprain or muscle strain. The normal rules of RICE apply: Rest (keep weight off the area); Ice it; keep inflammation down with Compression (a compression bandage); and Elevation (bring the affected area above the level of your heart).

COMMON PROBLEMS AND CULPRITS

The two major muscles that form the back of the calf, the gastrocnemius and, underneath it, the soleus, are the big guns of the lower leg. Although you generate most of your running power above the knee, from the quads and the hamstrings, the calf muscles add the final kick. Technically speaking, they are responsible for "plantar flexion"; that is, they pull the foot down away from the knee causing the foot to push off from the ground. The gastrocnemius and soleus run down the calf to form a common tendon, the massive Achilles tendon, which pulls up on the heel bone, transferring the pull of the two muscles. (Too much pressure on the tendon results in pain and inflammation. Achilles tendinitis is a common runner's complaint.) The antagonist muscles of the shin—tibialis anterior, extensor hallucis longus, and extensor digitorum longus—power the reverse action. That's "dorsiflexion"—lifting the toes up toward the knee.

The tendons of three lower-leg muscles run through a band of connective tissue on the inside of the ankle known as the tarsal tunnel. These "Tom, Dick, and Harry" tendons (*t*ibialis posterior, flexor *d*igitorum longus, and flexor *h*allucis longus) can press on or "impinge" the posterior tibial nerve inside the tunnel, causing inner ankle pain or numbness.

In a typical ankle sprain, the foot turns under and the outer part of the ankle rolls toward the ground. The peroneal muscles that run down the side of the leg stretch and tear, as does the anterior talofibular ligament on the outside of the joint.

The plantar fascia is a ligament made of a dense band of connective tissue that runs just underneath the sole, all the way from the heel to just behind the toes. It supports the major arch of the foot and facilitates the foot's movement. When the foot hits the ground too often or with too much force, the plantar fascia becomes painfully irritated (plantar fasciitis). The layers of muscle underneath it, including the flexor digitorum and the flexor hallucis brevis, often tighten up and contribute to the problem.

orthotic. Although we think orthotics can be overprescribed, for the right patient they can make a big difference. The art of treating the ankle/foot region, as with any hot spot, is knowing which treatment or combination of treatments suit the problem and when to use them. For feet problems, we often work in tandem with a talented Manhattan sports podiatrist (and triathlete), Dr. Dan Geller, who treats a number of the city's top runners and triathletes.

WHAT GOES WRONG, AND HOW TO FIX IT

Mostly Muscular

Plantar Fasciitis

Mike Llerandi, one of the country's top triathletes in his fortysomething age group, works fifty hours a week in the computer industry and trains thirty hours a week. Everything with him is on a tight schedule, and he couldn't afford a major disruption in his workout schedule if he was going to successfully compete in the Lake Placid triathalon. But less than two months before the race, Mike was hobbled with pain under the heel that extended down the arch of his foot—plantar fasciitis, a classic overuse injury. Dr. DeStefano manually treated the deep muscles of the foot underneath the plantar fascia, as well as the tight muscles in the calf that were pulling up too sharply on the heel, further irritating the area. Mike was getting better but not fast enough for the race. We sent him to sports podiatrist Dan Geller, who outfitted him with orthotics to take some of the pressure off the arch of the foot. Dr. Geller also gave him a corticosteroid injection to quiet the inflammation around the plantar fascia. Mike competed pain-free at Lake Placid and qualified for the Ironman triathalon in Hawaii. The foot and lower-leg exercises we gave him (see the end of the chapter) have kept him out of trouble since.

The feet take a constant pounding, especially from running. When the plantar fascia becomes irritated and inflamed, it's no joke. Whether it happens to a couch potato who takes up a little tennis or a hard-core endurance athlete such as Mike Llerandi, the symptoms are the same and often quite debilitating. The tight plantar fascia overstretches or slightly tears with every footfall, generating pain under the heel and sometimes down the arch. At night, the tissue contracts, so the first steps in the morning can be excruciating. The conventional medical advice is often ice and rest, which is fine, but as Mike Llerandi's case demonstrates, a lot more can be done to speed up healing. The key is not to focus just on the plantar fascia, the most obvious source of pain. We emptied out the toolbox for Mike— manual therapy to relieve tight foot and calf muscles that irritated the plantar fascia, orthotics to better support his high arches when standing or walking, and finally an anti-inflammatory injection. Another friend of ours, Olympic pentathlete Mike Gostigian (and also our male fitness model), came to us with what turned out to be a much easier case. His pain was so severe he had trouble walking, much less running with his training clients. But the plantar fascia was barely damaged. We loosened his calf muscles, which were pulling up on the heel, and he was fine.

Achilles Tendinitis

Jason ran the mile in high school. Considering he's in his midforties now, busy with family and career, it's been a while since he ran seriously. But he decided to get back in shape, so, being goal-oriented, he entered the New York City Marathon for extra motivation. Everything was going great until he amped up his training to over thirty miles a week and the Achilles tendon just above the back of his heel began to ache mercilessly every time he ran. He could feel the tightness in the back of his leg, so he figured stretching might help. It made things worse. When he got up in the morning, he couldn't even put weight on the affected leg. Dr. DeStefano steered clear of the Achilles tendon (Jason's stretching had only irritated it more), but working manually, he released muscular tension throughout the lower body. An obvious target were the two major calf muscles, which, in their tightened state, were pulling too hard on the tendon. He also loosened up the muscles in the foot, allowing them to soak up more running impact. Finally, he relaxed the tight muscles on the left side of the lower back, which had forced Jason's body to overcompensate by rotating too much to the right side. The result—Jason was landing harder on his right foot, the first link in a chain of imbalances that led to that overstressed right Achilles tendon. For Jason's part, he had to cut back on his training for a month to give his muscles and connective tissues a chance to adapt to the extra demands he was placing on them. He finished the marathon exhausted and sore but uninjured.

The Achilles tendon is the strongest tendon in the body, a massive cable linking calf muscles to heel bone. It's also the lower body's lightning rod for overuse injuries. As we saw with Jason, any combination of muscle tightness and imbalance can irritate the Achilles. Like a lot of people with Achilles tendinitis, he didn't help his cause by jumping into an aggressive sports program. Ideally, he should have prepared himself with muscle stretching and strengthening exercises (see the program at the end of this chapter), and the walk/run program we described in chapter 6. At a minimum, he needed to slowly build up his weekly mileage, making sure his system could handle the increasing load. Before every run, he should have warmed up for at least five or ten minutes with either a brisk walk or a slow jog. That increases blood flow to the muscles and tendons, loosening and warming them up. In collagen-based tendons, the tissue actually softens, reducing the chance it will be overstretched as it responds to the vigorous exercise to come. Our success with Jason, and a few thousand patients like him, has come from restoring balance and movement to the muscles that exert a force, directly or indirectly, on the Achilles tendon. If you're running with tense feet and stiff ankles, sooner or later you're going to have problems.

Achilles tendinitis is the lower body's version of tennis elbow (lateral epicondylitis). With overuse injuries, the overstressed tendons and surrounding muscle fibers microscopically tear and scar as they're repeatedly stretched out of shape. The *itis* in the name suggests that inflammation is at the root of the problem, but recent research tells us this usually isn't so. You might notice only a slight puffiness around that sore Achilles tendon. With chronic pain, what's often happening is that the collagen fibers have begun to deteriorate and become more vulnerable to further injury. (This is a condition more accurately called tendinosis.) Pain driven by tendonisis responds poorly to anti-inflammatories whether pills or injections.

SELF-DEFENSE

PROTECT YOUR FEET

Improperly fitted shoes can worsen muscle and tendon problems in the lower leg and foot, as well as cause calluses, bunions, and corns.

Make sure you've got the right athletic shoes for the job. For instance, cycling shoes should have rigid soles, running shoes softer, flexible soles, and all athletic shoes should be specific to the wearer's foot.

For chronic foot and leg problems, consider a shoe insert. You might want to start with over-the-counter arch supports, and if that doesn't solve the problem, try prescription orthotics. Inspect your old athletic shoes. If the inner edge of the soles is worn more heavily and, when you place them on a level surface, they tilt or collapse to the inside, you may be a good candidate for orthotics.

Run with relaxed feet and let the arches of the feet soak up impact shock. Running styles differ by individual, but, commonly, landing on the midfoot puts the least stress on the system.

(Plasma-enriched protein injections—see the box on page 129—may become a standard medical treatment for the most stubborn Achilles tendinitis cases.)

Muscle or Joint?

Tarsal Tunnel Syndrome

An area on the inner ankle called the tarsal tunnel can entrap the tibal nerve as it passes down into the foot, causing pain or sometimes numbness on the inside of the ankle. We can manually work to break up tightness in the muscles above the tarsal tunnel to get the tendons and the nerve to slide more smoothly against each other inside the fibrous-tissue tunnel. There is no one explanation for nerve impingement—it could be anything from a nerve cyst to a bone abnormality—so there is no one solution to the problem. In addition to muscle therapy, our patients have benefited from chiropractic extremity adjusting to take pressure off the joints, and also from anti-inflammatory injections.

Joint/Orthopedic

Ankle Sprain

When the New York Giants' Amani Toomer limped off the field during the last regular-season game of 2001, the team figured they had probably just lost their star wide receiver for the next week's play-off game. Amani had a serious sprain, but the MRI didn't show a tear in the anterior talofibular ligament (ATFL), the most vulnerable of the outer-ankle ligaments, which would definitely have kept him out. The team medical staff put him on crutches and immobilized the foot in a walking boot. The ankle was tender and swollen, but, with the athletic trainers, Dr. DeStefano was able to manually work on all the lower-leg muscles, especially the peroneals. By the end of the week, Amani was jogging. That Sunday, he caught a touchdown pass in the play-off victory against the Minnesota Vikings, which took the Giants to that year's Super Bowl.

Ankle sprains come with the territory. About three-quarters of ankle injuries are ankle sprains, the most common musculoskeletal injury in or out of sports. The foot rolls over, damaging the muscles and ligaments most commonly on the outside of the lower leg and ankle. The peroneal muscles are the first line of defense, then the ATFL. If all systems fail, you've got a foot fracture.

Ligaments heal on their own timetable, and if they tear, the body repairs them with collagen scar tissue, which means they'll be less supple and less strong than before the injury. As in Amani Toomer's case, the muscle component is usually a key to a speedy recovery. After a joint has been damaged, the body contracts the surrounding muscles to "splint" the area, limiting movement and reducing the chance for further injury. But after a couple of days, the joint has stabilized and the tight muscles actually impede healing. By manually releasing the tension in those lower-leg muscles, we can promote healing blood flow to the area and take pressure off the damaged joint. Severe ankle sprains may require surgery to repair the torn ligaments and stabilize the ankle.

Achilles Tendon Rupture

This one is a season-ender. In the typical scenario, a middle-aged recreational athlete, a tennis or a basketball player, shrugs off a chronically sore Achilles tendon. Over time, the collagen fibers of the tendon weaken, and blood flow to the area becomes compromised—the tendinosis that sets the stage for serious injury. All it takes is one forceful lunge and the tendon completely rips from the bone. You may hear a popping sound; you may feel as if someone has kicked you in the heel. If it really is a full rupture, you won't be able to stand on your toes. The usual remedy, at least for anyone who wants to return to sports and an active lifestyle, is surgery to reattach the tendon.

We have had professional athletes suffer complete Achilles tendon ruptures who, after we've worked on their muscles before and after surgery, come back the next year 100 percent.

Morton's Neuroma

In probably the most common nerve disorder in the foot, the digital nerve that runs between the toes becomes compressed, causing a sharp or burning pain, usually between the third and the fourth toes. Tight women's shoes with narrow toeboxes are the usual culprits. Switching to shoes with a wider toebox (possibly with a pad underneath the ball of each foot) and a lower heel is the first step. Manual therapy on the muscles of the forefoot can sometimes relieve the pressure on the nerve; sometimes a corticosteroid injection does the job. When all else fails, the nerve is surgically cut, eliminating the pain, and all sensation, in the area.

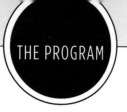

ANKLE/FOOT

The muscles of the lower leg play a huge role in gait, stabilization of the lower extremities, and other movement patterns of the lower body. They can also be the source of dysfunction that works its way through the movement chains into other areas of the body. A healthy posture and gait are dependent on the proper function of the ankle and the foot.

ANTERIOR LOWER LEG

Purpose: To target and remove restrictions and restore a full range of motion to the tibialis anterior by manually releasing tight, short, and damaged muscles.

Starting out: Sit on the floor with one leg straight and the treatment leg bent with the heel on the floor and the toes pulled up and back. Using both hands, place your thumbs over the muscle with angled pressure up toward the knee. The two treatment zones are the inside (closer to the shinbone) and outside aspects of the tibialis anterior.

How to do it: Press in and pull up slightly, as though trying to prevent someone from sliding a piece of cloth from under your fingers. Maintaining angled pressure, point your toe and extend the ankle. Repeat with your other leg. Do two to three passes, releasing and moving the hand from the knee toward the foot, in each zone.

Troubleshooting: Don't press too hard as this can irritate the muscles. Avoid letting your skin slide under the fingers by using angled pressure.

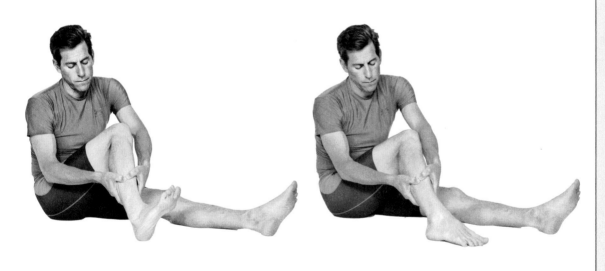

LATERAL LOWER LEG

Purpose: To target and remove restrictions and restore a full range of motion to the peroneal group by manually releasing tight, short, and damaged muscles.

Starting out: Sit on the floor with one leg straight and the treatment leg bent. Place the outside of the treatment heel on the floor, with your ankle straight and your foot angled out to the side. Using both hands, place your thumbs over the muscle with angled pressure. The treatment zone is a small strip on the side of the leg between the tibialis anterior and the calf.

How to do it: Press in and pull up slightly, as though trying to prevent someone from sliding a piece of cloth from under your fingers. Maintaining angled pressure, flex the ankle and twist the foot in, bringing the outside edge of the foot toward the floor. Repeat with your other leg. Do two to three passes, releasing and moving your hand, from the knee toward the foot.

Troubleshooting: Don't press too hard as this can irritate the muscles. Avoid letting the skin slide under your fingers by using angled pressure.

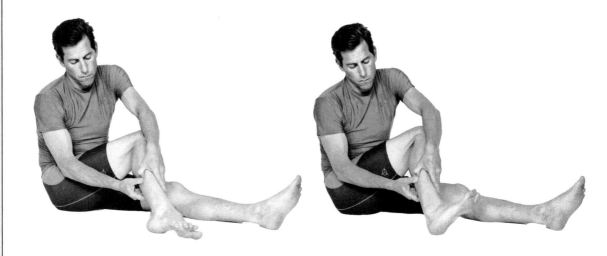

SOLE OF THE FOOT

Purpose: To target dysfunction, irritation, and inflammation in the plantar fascia by releasing the fascia and muscles and icing involved tissues.

Starting out: Sit on a stability ball or chair with your feet shoulders' width apart. The arch of the treatment foot should rest on a small, ribbed plastic bottle of frozen water. The movement should start with the foot curved over and pressed slightly into the bottle.

How to do it: Press in and forward slightly with the foot and pull the toes back and as far up as is comfortable. Repeat with the other foot. Do two to three passes, releasing and moving the position of the bottle from the toes toward the heel.

Troubleshooting: Don't press too hard as this can irritate the muscles. Keep the body balanced on the ball so the treatment foot does not also have to work to balance.

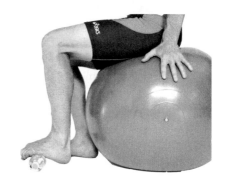

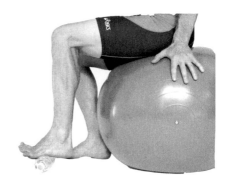

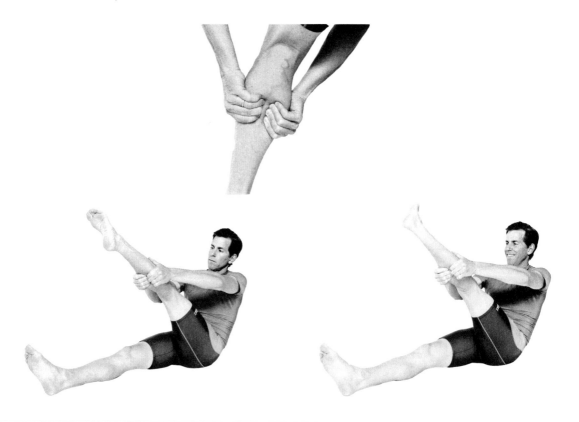

POSTERIOR LOWER LEG
A. GASTROCNEMIUS

Purpose: To target and remove restrictions and restore a full range of motion to the posterior lower leg—especially the gastrocnemius—by releasing tight, short, and damaged muscles.

Starting out: Sit on the floor with the treatment leg bent and the foot on the floor. Your other leg should be extended for balance. Your hands should be wrapped around the treatment leg so that the fingers contact the calf muscles and your thumbs stabilize on the front of the leg. The toes should be pointed and the knee slightly bent. The three treatment zones are the inside, middle, and outside portions of the back of the lower leg.

How to do it: Press in and pull up slightly, creating angled pressure, then straighten your knee and pull the toes up toward your nose. Repeat with your other leg. Do two to three passes, releasing and moving the hand position from a third of the way up the calf toward the knee, in each of the zones.

Troubleshooting: Don't press too hard as this can irritate the muscles. Keep the body relaxed and balanced, so your focus can be on the treatment.

S E L F - T R E A T M E N T • S T R E T C H E S • E X E R C I S E S •

B. SOLEUS AND ACHILLES TENDON

Purpose: To target and remove restrictions and restore a full range of motion to the posterior lower leg—especially the soleus and the Achilles tendon—by releasing tight, short, and damaged muscles.

Starting out: Sit on the floor with one leg straight and the treatment leg bent with your heel on the floor and the toes pointed. Your hands should be wrapped around the treatment leg so that the fingers contact the calf muscles and the thumbs stabilize on the front of the leg. The three treatment zones are the inside, middle, and outside portions of the leg.

How to do it: Press in and pull up slightly, creating angled pressure, while pulling the toes toward the nose. Repeat with your other leg. Do two to three passes in each zone, releasing and moving the position of the hands from the ankle toward the knee. You don't have to extend the knee because this muscle doesn't cross the joint. Also, it extends lower down the leg than the gastrocnemius.

Troubleshooting: Don't press too hard as this can irritate the muscles. Keep the body relaxed and balanced, so your focus can be on the treatment.

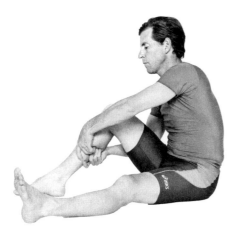 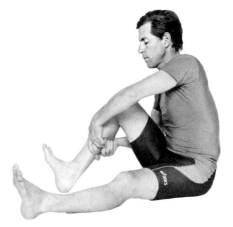

ANTERIOR LOWER LEG AND LATERAL LOWER LEG

Purpose: To lengthen the tibialis anterior, the deep muscles and tendons of the anterolateral lower leg, and the muscles of the top of the foot.

Starting out: Stand with all your weight balanced on one leg and the foot of the treatment leg gently placed on the floor behind the first leg with the toes curled under.

How to do it: Slowly put some body weight on the treatment foot, gently rolling forward onto the backs of the toes in a pain-free range of motion. Hold the stretch for two seconds, then return to the starting position. Repeat with your other foot. Repeat ten times.

Variation: With the toes rolled under, bring the heel out to the side. This will stretch the side of the foot and the peroneals.

Troubleshooting: Don't just compress the toes under the body's weight. Roll the toes in a curling motion until a stretch is felt in the anterior leg. Actively curling the toes is the best way to enhance this stretch.

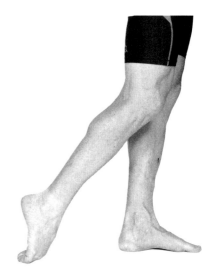

PLANTAR FASCIA AND POSTERIOR LOWER LEG

Purpose: To lengthen the muscles of the gastrocnemius, soleus, Achilles tendon, and plantar fascia.

Starting out: Stand upright with one leg forward and the treatment leg back, about two feet from heel to toe, or whatever distance enables you to feel a stretch. The heel of the treatment leg should be raised to relax the muscle.

How to do it: Lower the heel so that the treatment leg is straight and lean forward until a gentle stretch is felt in the back of the lower leg. This stretch should be held for two to three seconds, returning to the starting position after each rep. Repeat ten times. Go immediately into the second part of the stretch from the same starting position. Lower the heel and sit back into the treatment leg in a controlled manner until a deeper, gentle stretch is felt in the posterior lower leg. Hold the stretch for two seconds, returning to the starting position after each rep. Repeat ten times. Repeat both parts of the stretch with your other leg.

Troubleshooting: Do not rush these stretches or push them to the point of pain. Slow, relaxed, and controlled motions are the best way to develop length in this complex of muscles.

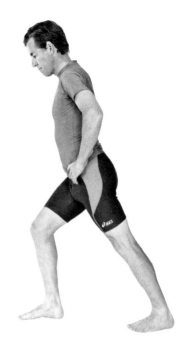

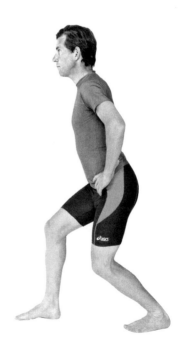

POSTERIOR LOWER LEG AND LATERAL LOWER LEG

Purpose: To lengthen the muscle/movement chain from the plantar fascia up the leg through the calf and even into the hamstrings.

Starting out: Sit on a chair with one foot on the floor for stability and the treatment leg partially extended. Your knee should be slightly bent and the foot relaxed. Hold a rope looped around the ball of the foot, just at the base of the toes.

How to do it: Straighten the leg and simultaneously pull the toes back with the foot and the foot back with the rope. This should gently stretch the back of the leg, ankle, and sole of the foot. Hold the stretch for two seconds, then return to the starting position. Repeat with your other leg. Repeat ten times.

Variation: With the foot flexed, pivot the bottom of the foot from one side to the other to stretch the inside and the outside of the ankle and calf.

Troubleshooting: Don't roll the body forward to meet the leg—keep the abs engaged and maintain a straight posture. Pull with your arms; don't lean back to pull the rope.

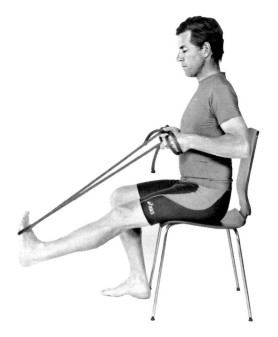

ANTERIOR LOWER LEG AND LATERAL LOWER LEG

Purpose: Toe pulls with a flex-band to strengthen the muscles of the anterior and lateral leg. This helps with gait, posture, and stability.

Starting out: Sit on a chair with your feet shoulders' width apart. A flex-band should be fixed around the nontreatment foot, then stretched at a tension appropriate to your ability across to the treatment foot. It should be looped around the ball of the treatment foot, with the free end held out of the way. The bottom of the treatment foot should be slightly contracted so the outside edge of the ball of the foot and the little toe rest on the floor.

How to do it: Roll your foot against the flex-band's resistance so that the foot ends up on the inside edge. To do this, simultaneously lift the toes, roll the foot, and lift the outside edge of the foot. Repeat with your other foot. Do ten repetitions, held for no more than two seconds each.

Troubleshooting: Remember to return to the starting position and relax between each repetition. Remember to include both parts of the movement—don't just raise your foot. Stay relaxed but balanced. Only the feet should be active; the rest of your body stays neutral.

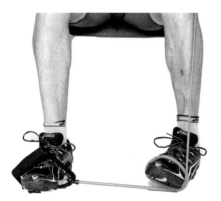
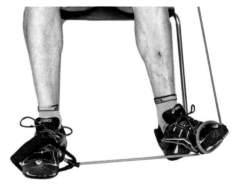

PLANTAR FASCIA

Purpose: Towel grasp and pull to strengthen the muscles of the foot and the articulation of the toes. This helps with gait, posture, and arch weakness. This also warms up the muscles and helps prevent strain on other structures of the body.

Starting out: Sit on a stability ball or chair with your feet shoulders' width apart. Place one foot on the ground for stability and the ball of the treatment foot on a towel or cloth. The towel should be weighted with a book or other object with enough weight to create resistance. If the exercise is too difficult with the book, try it without any weight.

How to do it: Pull your toes in, trying to grasp the towel and gather it up under the foot. Repeat with your other foot. Do ten repetitions, held for no more than two seconds each.

Troubleshooting: Stay relaxed but balanced on the ball, so that the focus can be on the treatment foot. Do not move your heel; simply flex the toes to grab the towel.

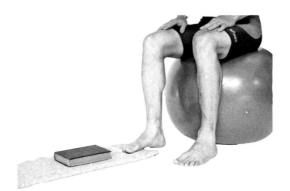 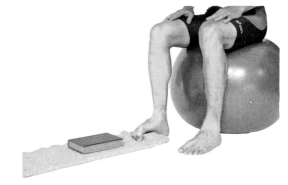

PLANTAR FASCIA AND POSTERIOR LOWER LEG

Purpose: Toe raisers to strengthen the muscles of the foot and the calf. This helps with gait, posture, and arch weakness. This also warms up the muscles and helps prevent strain on other structures of the body.

Starting out: Stand with your feet shoulders' width apart, with your weight balanced between your toes and heels.

How to do it: Shift your weight to your toes and raise the heels off the floor, lifting as high up onto the toes as is possible. Do ten repetitions, held for no more than two seconds each.

Troubleshooting: Keep the body relaxed but balanced; do not lean forward or look down. Only the feet should be active; the rest of the body stays neutral.

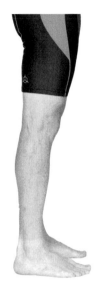

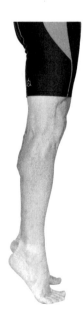

SUMMARY AND EPILOGUE

Maybe you're familiar with the Indian fable about the blind travelers who come across an elephant in the road. One man feels the trunk, another a tusk, another the flank, and the last one, the tail. As you might guess, they arrive at very different conclusions about what that elephant looks like. The way that Western medicine treats musculoskeletal problems is something like that: trauma surgeons look at the body and see bones that need to be fixed, sports medicine orthopedists see joints that need repair, chiropractors want to mobilize joints, muscle therapists want to work directly on the muscles, and physical therapists want to strengthen the muscles and make them more flexible. Between these groups, they've got that elephant pretty well covered, but they all need to work together!

As we've often said, to understand injuries and treat them effectively, you've got to deal with the whole elephant—bone, joint, and muscle. Ignore one or two of the elements and you could miss the big picture. Recall the soccer player in chapter 1 who tore his ACL: classic sports injury, textbook surgery, and yet he didn't really attain the full benefit until Dr. DeStefano addressed the muscle damage in his thigh in rehab. Or the businesswoman marathoner we discussed in chapter 12. Dr. DeStefano won her some symptomatic relief by manually treating the muscles, but she wasn't really going to get better until Dr. Kelly surgically dealt with both bone (the impaired mobility in the hip socket) and joint (torn hip cartilage).

By now we hope you appreciate the importance of muscle in the overall health-care puzzle. And beyond that, how important it is to treat a musculoskeletal problem in the proper sequence. First, tight, damaged muscles have to be addressed and the body's healing process mobilized. Then we move on to muscle conditioning—stretching and strengthening. That's how we work with our patients, and that's how you will work on yourself when using our self-help program. That, in sum, is muscle medicine, a philosophy about how the musculoskeletal system works and a strategy for treating it.

In this final chapter, we're going to do two things. First, we'll quickly summarize the tools for healthy living that we offer throughout the book. Then we'll present a guide for skillfully using these tools in the real world; in other words, how to be the smartest consumer of musculoskeletal health care—muscle therapy and surgery—that you can be.

MUSCLE MEDICINE REVIEW

Chapter 2 explained the basic biology of how your muscles, joints, and bones work together as an integrated system. Chapter 3 went deeper into how this system commonly breaks down. When you're dealing with an injury, it's easy to get bogged down in the Latinate names that your doctor might be tossing at you—*patellofemoral syndrome* or *iliotibial band syndrome,* for instance. You should know that there are many of the same underlying causes behind the different muscle problems that we discuss. Appreciating that will help you talk intelligently with your doctor, or to do your own online research.

Chapter 4 addressed the psychological dimension of injuries. Self-awareness is the tool to reduce your own contribution to physical wear and tear. Everyday stress can cause your muscles to tighten up. So can fear about a physical or medical issue that you don't adequately understand. All these things can feed into a cycle of distress and pain.

Chapter 5 was a general introduction to good nutrition. The right diet is an important part of maintaining a healthy musculoskeletal system, and for many readers weight loss is crucial. The simple truth about weight loss is: eat less, exercise more. The number of calories you consume must be less than the number you expend.

Chapter 6 offered some ideas about smart and effective exercising in an all-around fitness program broad enough for almost anyone to use as a guide. If you're unsure of any of the advice in this chapter, seek out a qualified personal trainer to teach you the basics of good form and how to construct a balanced exercise program. The trainer should be willing to work with you to achieve your fitness goals, and with any health professional involved in your care.

Chapter 8 through 14 dealt with what we call the hot spots. The chapters discussed in detail some of the most common musculoskeletal problems occurring in the neck, the shoulder, the elbow, wrist, and hand, the lower back, the hip, the knee, and the ankle/foot. In these chapters, we went from discussing what a therapist or an M.D. can do for you to what you can do for yourself. And at the end of each hot-spot chapter, you were shown the muscle medicine self-help program, which moves, in logical sequence, from muscle self-treatment to stretching to strength work.

As we explained in chapter 7, the introduction to the self-help program, many treatments exist to manually address tight and damaged muscles, including chiropractic, acupuncture, physical therapy, as well as hands-on techniques such as ART and Trigger Point Therapy. We've applied elements of these techniques to create our method of self-treatment that you can effectively do yourself. For the stretching and strength work—the conditioning part of our self-help program—we've tried to distill the best of the best from the exercises that health professionals give their clients and patients.

If you are ready to move from a doctor or a therapist's care, discuss with your doctor whether our self-help program would be safe and helpful for you. We've designed it to work for a broad collection of people: people in good health; people with minor musculoskeletal problems that don't interfere with their everyday activities; people with more serious problems who have been cleared by their physicians to supplement professional care with this program; and for people who have been through treatment for more serious conditions and now, posttherapy or postsurgery, have been cleared by their doctor to continue to work on their health with this program.

BEING AN EDUCATED HEALTH-CARE CONSUMER: CONTRACTORS VS. SUBCONTRACTORS

It's important to have a good foundation of musculoskeletal self-knowledge. In today's fragmented health-care system, you're going to need it to be a smart health-care consumer. Let's take the first decision you face when a chronic problem surfaces or you suffer a trauma (one that doesn't send you to the emergency room): whom do you call?

We can make this decision less daunting by making a simple comparison. Imagine that searching out musculoskeletal health care is like building a house or undertaking major renovations. You can find a contractor you trust and leave the major decisions to him. Or you can play that role yourself and search out the subcontractors you think are best equipped to handle the many jobs involved in your project (lay the foundation, handle the electrical, and so on). In the case of serious joint injury, the orthopedist will most likely serve as your contractor. An alternative is a physiatrist or an osteopathic physician (D.O.). These days, osteopathy has many functions—drugs are prescribed, surgeries are performed—but the profession's roots are in manual manipulation, and some D.O.'s combine conventional medicine with hands-on expertise. If your problem has more to do with muscle or nerves (a backache or a sore wrist from overusing the keyboard), a chiropractor could make a first-rate contractor.

The contractor may be calling most of the shots, but of course the onus is on you to find the right one! Let's consider the search for an orthopedist to manage a joint injury. It's likely that your primary-care doctor will refer you to someone. That's a start, but it doesn't have to be the final word. Talk to your friends and colleagues. Is someone particularly satisfied with their surgically replaced knee, or dissatisfied? Web research can be helpful. To begin, check out www.bestdoctors.com and the Web site for the American Academy of Orthopaedic Surgeons (www.aaos.org). You might want to talk to any college or professional sport teams in your area and find out which surgeons they entrust their athletes to. The same holds true when you're searching out manual therapists.

As you narrow your list of candidates for surgeons, take a closer look at their résumés. Where did they intern? Do they have teaching responsibilities? The hospital and the surgeon you settle on should routinely perform the procedure you are

● Dr. DeStefano

I had a patient, a female runner, with terrible groin pain. I treated her for weeks and weeks and she only got moderate relief. But she was convinced that the problem was muscular. Finally, I persuaded her to get an MRI of her hip, and it came back negative. I treated her some more. She got a second MRI at an MRI center that was covered by her insurance, but it didn't have the best reputation. Again, negative. Finally, I persuaded her to go to the Hospital for Special Surgery and pay half the cost out of pocket. They found an impinged hip and an absolutely shredded labral cartilage. The difference in quality between radiology centers can be amazing. Dr. Kelly cleaned out the joint and repaired it. My patient is back to running, pain-free, and it had much more to do with the joint than the muscle!

considering, many times a week, if not every day. Practice makes perfect. Just how high you need to set the bar for your prospective surgeon depends on the procedure you're in the market for. Minimally invasive surgery to repair a torn labrum cartilage in the hip is a new field. You want a leader in that field, not someone who does the operation occasionally. But even for something as seemingly straightforward as an ACL reconstruction, different types of procedures must be considered. Do your research!

When you choose an orthopedist, the doctor should be ready to enter into a working partnership. It's not an equal relationship—the orthopedist knows more about orthopedics than you do—but the right doctor and support staff can help educate you with printed materials on surgical procedures and tips on how to find reliable information on the Web. The Web site for the Hospital for Special Surgery (www.hss.edu), for instance, is packed with downloadable instructional videos for most any orthopedic procedure you could imagine.

Beyond the technical ABC's, an orthopedist should provide straight talk. What functional gains can realistically be expected from this surgery? How does that stack up against the costs: the risks on the operating table; the time lost at work or at home; the length and difficulty of the rehab. Sometimes what patients fail to grasp is that the goal of the surgery may be a joint that works *better* than it did before surgery, not one that works perfectly.

Finally, your best surgeon may be the one who chooses *not* to operate. Any board-certified orthopedist can do a procedure. But it takes experience, and the judgment that comes with it, to know when not to operate. In the hot-spot chapters, you've seen cases where surgery was a plausible, maybe even expected, solution to a musculoskeletal problem, but in our view it wasn't the best option at that time. Especially in areas where judgment calls can be toughest—a piece of torn meniscus cartilage in the knee, a herniated disk in the lumbar spine—you want an orthopedist who is secure in his practice and in his conservative judgment. Even when due diligence has paid off and you've found such a surgeon, as a rule of thumb, you should get a second, possibly even a third opinion, before deciding to go forward with a procedure. Orthopedic surgery can work wonders, but all potential options should be explored.

HOW TO MANAGE YOUR DOCTOR OR THERAPIST

Dealing with injury can be emotional and disorienting. To get the most benefit from a visit to the orthopedist to discuss treatment options, bring a friend or family member as a more objective "second set of ears." Have the person take notes or tape-record the visit.

Bring a list of no more than five important questions to ask. Talk to the doctor's support staff about the smaller stuff such as, "Where can I get an ice pack?"

Don't get frustrated by a quick visit. What you don't see is the doctor reviewing your chart, studying your X-rays or MRIs, talking about your case with colleagues. The time you actually spend in his office is just the tip of the iceberg, usually a time for assessment, not for treatment.

E-mail is a great way to communicate with your doctors. That way they can respond to you when they have an available moment rather than try to coordinate two busy schedules for a phone call.

In therapy, you should not be left unattended on an exercise machine or a device. The therapist should be focused on you, not trying to take care of multiple patients at once. If that's the situation, find a more suitable therapy program and be willing to pay out of pocket for it. Your body is worth it.

SEARCHING OUT THE SUBCONTRACTORS

As we said earlier, for less severe musculoskeletal injuries, it may not be necessary or even desirable to put yourself in the hands of one practitioner and have him or her make all the big decisions. Here, you may want to assume the role of contractor and investigate a range of therapies, and perhaps even put together a package of therapies to address different aspects of the same problem. Perhaps your physician suggests acupuncture, but you're afraid of needles. You might want to look into acupressure or Trigger Point Therapy, where pressure from a therapist's thumbs and fingers may achieve a similar effect.

Good research is the key. Go back to our brief discussion of manual therapies in chapter 7 for a starting point, then follow up online. Established muscle therapies such as ART (www.activerelease.com), Graston Technique (www.grastontechnique.com), Myofascial Release (www.myofascialrelease.com), Orthopedic Massage (www.orthomassage.net), and Trigger Point Therapy (www.triggerpointbook.com), and many others are all well represented on the Web. Sometimes the particular school of therapy is less important than finding a skilled therapist who works in your area. Word of mouth can often lead you to that person.

What should you look for during that first visit with a muscle therapist? To begin with, you and the therapist should agree on a clear plan of action. First, how does the therapist intend to get you out of pain? Then, how will he or she try to find the source of the pain and fix the problem? Is there a plan for occasional maintenance visits or advice on prevention strategies so that the problem does not return? Ideally, you will have exercises to do on your own time to continue treatment at home. Most manual muscle therapy (as opposed to chiropractic and physical therapy rehabilitation and conditioning) is not covered by insurance, so plan accordingly for out-of-pocket costs.

The therapist should be able to give you a rough idea of how many sessions may be required to resolve or improve your muscle issue. Obviously, a lot depends on how entrenched and complicated the muscle injury is. Some problems can be resolved in a single session, some may take weeks of treatment. If you're not seeing positive results after three or four sessions, you should discuss it with your therapist and possibly reconsider your choice of treatment. This doesn't mean that the therapy doesn't work, only that it or the therapist is not a good match for your particular problem.

THE TEAM CONCEPT

You should always look for a muscle therapist who can see the big picture and identify issues outside of his or her scope. The therapist should have collegial relationships with other types of health-care providers and the experience to recognize, for instance, when a painful joint should be looked at by an orthopedist, or some other specialist if an underlying medical condition is suspected (a tumor? diabetes?). Maybe a physical therapist should be brought in to strengthen weak muscles if that is what's holding back recovery. A chiropractor can treat joint misalignments.

As you can tell, we strongly believe in the team concept—our own collaboration has taught us that every therapy or treatment has an important role to play. For instance, if diet and weight are troubling issues, see a nutritionist. A knowledgeable trainer can inject real value into a gym membership and play a crucial role in helping clients with the transition from a structured physical therapy program to working out at the gym.

It's true that not every talented health-care practitioner is a team player. Your surgeon, for instance, may have formidable technical skills but not be very engaged in your postsurgical rehab. You could wind up in a "cookie-cutter" physical therapy program that offers little individual attention and no manual therapy expertise because your insurance doesn't cover it. Then it's your responsibility to find a surgeon or physical therapist who meets your standards and be willing to pay out of pocket for it.

To take an example from the manual therapy world, let's suppose you're getting great results with a traditional acupuncturist who lives and breathes only acupuncture. That's fine, but now it's your responsibility to seek out the appropriate care for any problem that falls outside that particular skill set. If the therapist sends out the signal, subtly or not so subtly, that going outside his or her method for a complementary treatment, or even just a second opinion, is not acceptable, find another therapist. For that matter, if a surgeon discourages you from seeking a second opinion, that's a bad sign as well. But don't confuse that with the orthopedist who holds you back from jumping into an exercise program or the muscle therapist who cautions you about making a fast decision about surgery. They're respecting the body's healing time line, not rejecting other styles of care.

By now, you've seen the limitations of a system in which health problems are treated by separate groups of specialists who sometimes don't have much contact with one another. The body isn't an inanimate object like a car that you can drop off at one shop to get the dents knocked out and at another to get the brakes fixed, and then pick it up expecting it to work without a hitch. The body is a living organism. All the moving parts affect one another; all aspects need to be considered. That's why we believe in a flexible team approach to deal with the range of musculo-skeletal problems, from mostly muscular to mostly joint. We have plans to open a hip center where the best talents—orthopedics, manual therapists, and physical therapists—are all collected under one roof. We hope it will be a model that others find useful. This book is just a first step.

● Dr. Kelly

I am just as happy, if not happier, when someone comes in for surgery and I can say, "I don't think that is the way to go. Let's deal with the muscle." They're usually skeptical. They'll say, "I've been dealing with this for so long. I just want it fixed." And I have to say, "Be a little patient. Trust me on this one." And I'll send them to Dr. DeStefano. My approach is not trying to be a surgeon so much as a health-care professional—trying to figure out the best solution to the problem. And I don't want to do surgery on people if they're not going to do well. Maybe 10 percent of patients don't do so well, but they take up 90 percent of my time—"I'm still not getting better, what's wrong?" That's painful to hear. And that's a strong incentive for a surgeon to help people get better without surgery if they can.

ACKNOWLEDGMENTS

DR. ROBERT DeSTEFANO

So many things have to come together in order to write a book that it seems impossible to individually acknowledge and adequately thank everyone who has had a part in this enormous undertaking. If we have missed anyone, we are truly sorry.

Thank you to all of my patients who have supported me over the past twenty-five years and entrusted me with their health, as well as the health of their family members, friends, and colleagues. A special thanks to Ms. Carolyn Reidy for her encouragement and support of this project from the beginning and throughout the process. Thank you to Dr. Bryan Kelly, whose vision allows him to help his patients completely: both through his amazing talent as a surgeon and his incorporation of other health care professionals.

To Susan Stanley: partner, friend, scholar, and exceptional manual therapist. Without her help, this book would not have gotten done. Thank you.

To Joe Hooper for putting our thoughts into a simple, meaningful manuscript that people can understand. Thanks to his wife, Kate, for her help. To Michael Gostigian and his family for help on so many levels: thank you for modeling for the book, for representing our country in three consecutive Olympic Games as a modern pentathalete, for contributing to the fitness section, for keeping me aware of the importance of exercise, for so many referrals to our offices, and for teaching those around you to live life fully by your example and not just words. Most of all, thanks for your friendship. Thanks to Megan Fanslau for modeling for the book and her help in the office, which she always gave with a smile. Thanks to Zach Schisgal for a wonderful job of editing and coordinating this book, and for helping to make it a reality. Special thanks to Shawna Lietzke, for always being there to answer questions, and for all of her hard work. Thanks to Mike Llerandi for his friendship, advice, and contributions to this book. Thanks to Eric and Brooke Lagstein at Be Creative Photography for their contributions and pictures. Their expertise and advice were priceless.

Thank you to my children, Jason, Amy, and Julie, who teach me the most about life and keep me honest and true. You are everything to me. To Gayle, their mother, for her tireless commitment to and care of our children. Thanks to my family for everything, especially my mother and father for their love and support and for bringing me into this beautiful world.

Thank you to all of my friends and family who supported this book, and my fellow professionals and colleagues who so generously help others. To Dr. Mike Leahy, creator of Active Release Techniques, and his family: thank you for the opportunity to help others and for opening my mind to the treatment of muscles and their role in health care. Thanks to Dr. Janet Travel—so far ahead of her time—and Dr. David Simmons for the work they've pioneered in the field of Trigger Point Therapy. To Dr. John Mennel and his manual manipulation expertise, and Dr. Raymond Nimmo—a true inspiration.

Thank you to Dr. Russell Warren, Dr. Scott Rodeo, and all of the physicians at the Hospital for Special Surgery. To Dr. Jen Solomon, Dr. Frank Lipman, Dr. Marc Polimeni, Dr. Kenneth Conti, Dr. Dan Geller, Dr. Marcus Forman, Deanie Barth, MSPT, and Dr. Lisa Callahan: thank you for your referrals and confidence.

Thanks to Ronnie Barnes for teaching me the most valuable lesson of my career: to be a piece of the treatment puzzle when working with a team of medical professionals in an integrative setting. To Byron Hansen, Steve Kennelly, Leigh Weiss, and the New York Giants' athletic training staff. To Joe and Ed Skiba, Ed Wagner, Tim Slaman, and all of the New York Giants' equipment room staff.

Thanks to the Mara and Tisch families for giving me the opportunity to serve such a professionally run organization—the New York Football Giants. And to Coach Coughlin, and all the Giants' coaching staff.

Thank you to all of the New York Football Giants players who I have helped over the years, and who have supported me and value the treatment I provide. There are too many to list, but special thanks to Jeff Feagles, Amani Toomer,

Michael Strahan, Eli Manning, Tiki Barber, Chase Blackburn, David Diehl, Antonio Pierce, and Howard Cross.

Thanks to Chris and Katy Gebhardt and family, to Dr. Marvin and Wendy Lagstein and family, Howard and Pia Cross and family, the Llerandi family, George and Brooke Perez and family, Darren Prince and family, Dr. Mark Delmonte and family, Tom LaTorre and family, James Carr, Esq., and family, and Dr. Bob Zimmerman—all of whom inspire, challenge, and motivate me.

Thanks to Harlan Schlecter, Geri and Kit Laybourne, Natalie Moody, Mr. John Tishman, Donald Schupak, and Sister Carol Zinn—my mentors and guides through life.

Thanks to Pat Manocchia for the opportunity to work with him, his clients, and his staff, and to learn and share in a truly innovative, integrative environment. Thank you to the Manocccchia family. Thanks to all at La Palestra who have helped me in so many ways over the last ten years, especially Greg Peters, Shannon Plumstead, Mark Tenore, Kofi Sekyiamah, Mike Pardo and family, and Greg Cimino, for his constant and expert legal advice on all of my projects.

Thank you to all my associates and office staff over the years, especially Dr. Kyler Brown, Dr. Keren Day, Dr. Justina Ngo, Dr. Andrew Veech, and Dr. Marie-Claude Goyette, as well as Kathy Salcedo and all the staff who have assisted me to help our patients and keep our offices running smoothly.

Thanks to Phil and Jim Wharton for opening my eyes to the importance of the right stretch at the right time, and to Joe Brown and Vincent Guida for helping me to create the FAST Stick.

Thanks to my Active Release Techniques friends, colleagues, and instructors. There are too many to mention, but special thanks to Dr. Tony Criscuolo, Dr. Joe Pelino, Dr. Tammara Moore, Jan Wanklyn, LMT, Dr. Gerry Ramogida, Dr. Dale Buchberger, Dr. Lawrence Micheli, and all of my fellow instructors. Thank you for your support and friendship over the years.

Palmer College of Chiropractic—the Fountainhead. Thank you for a great profession and the opportunity to help others. Thanks to Palmer Rugby and Eric Seiler for allowing me to represent the Palmer Rugby Club.

To Kutztown University, New York Chiropractic College, and Phil Santiago for helping me in the field of Sports Chiropractic. Thanks to Ridgefield Park High

School for starting me on the journey by introducing me to basic science. Thank you to Bill Weber for getting me started. Thanks to Dr. John Piazza for your motivation and energy!

Thank you to the sport of triathlon, USA Triathlon, World Triathlon Corporation, North American Sports, Gram Fraser and family, and Shelley Bramblett and family. Thank you to Jim Brown, Joe Branda, Rich Byrne, Frank Guadagnino, and all my coaches throughout the years.

Thank you to all the athletes I've treated over the years from many different sports: Mike Kahn and the Olympic bobsled program; the Olympic skeleton and luge team; Cami Granato and the women's U.S. hockey team; world championship skaters Adam Rippon, Miki Ando, and Anna Zadorozhniuk; NBA players and administration; and NHL players and administration. Thanks to SAG and all my friends in the entertainment industry. Special thanks to those who endorsed this book: John McEnroe, Cristie Kerr, Natalie Gulbis, Elisabeth Hasselbeck, and Liam Neeson.

Thank you, the reader, for choosing this book and trusting us to help you to help yourself.

DR. BRYAN KELLY

First and foremost, I would like to acknowledge my loving wife, Lois, and our beautiful children, Conor, Emma, and Jack. I would also like to acknowledge my father, mother, and brother. Without all of their love and support I would never have been able to accomplish what I have thus far in my career. Taking care of patients and athletes can have a huge impact on your family life. Injuries often occur at inconvenient times, and caring for these injuries may force time away from home. Without an understanding core group that supports one's desire to treat these injuries, it would be an impossible and thankless job. With their endless support, one can truly experience the satisfaction of getting patients back to full function and mobility.

Second, I would like to acknowledge the two clinicians in the field of Orthopaedics and Sports Medicine that have had the greatest impact on my career and practice—Dr. Russell F. Warren and Ronnie P. Barnes. Dr. Warren and Mr. Barnes have worked together for more than twenty-five years as the head team physician and head athletic trainer for the New York Football Giants. They have shown me the true importance and value of working collaboratively to provide better patient care as a team than can ever be provided as individuals. They embody the underlying spirit of this book—the immeasurable importance of integrating different approaches to provide a more comprehensive and successful treatment plan for the patients and athletes that we care for. Both have been an invaluable source of pure clinical knowledge and experience that will forever affect the way that I think about athletic injury and treatment. There is not a day that goes by in my practice that I do not try to imagine how these icons of Sports Medicine would think about a particular clinical problem.

Finally, I would like to acknowledge my patients, who have been a constant source of both satisfaction and frustration, but have always been the source of continued learning and experience. I was taught in my training that if you listen carefully to your patients, they will tell you the answer to their problems, and in many cases offer you the correct solution. It is amazing how intuitive patients are about their own injury, and the art of listening and reacting to the information that they provide is something that can never be overemphasized.

JOE HOOPER

My first and deepest thanks go to my mentors in "muscle medicine," Rob DeStefano and Bryan Kelly, to massage therapist Sue Stanley, whose late-in-the-game editing and writing contributions made finishing this book possible, and to my wife, Kate Doyle Hooper, who kept me sane throughout. I also owe a debt of gratitude to an all-star team of friends and colleagues whose generously shared expertise allowed us to dare to cover so much ground: sports podiatrist Dan Geller; trainer (and fitness model) extraordinaire Mike Gostigian; triathlete and fitness authority Mike Llerondi; physical therapist Toni McGinley; nutritionist Heidi Skolnik; and physiatrist Jen Solomon. Valuable contributions were also made by physical therapist Deanie Barth, muscle therapist/chiropractor Keren Day, ergonomist Ellen Kolber, integrative physician Frank Lipman, neurosurgeon Ted Schwartz, and stretching "guru" Jim Wharton. How we have assimilated their ideas into this book is, of course, the sole responsibility of the authors.

INDEX

Page numbers in *italics* refer to illustrations.

hand:
    numbness in, 127
    overuse injuries of, 125
    versatility of, 126
    see also elbow/wrist/hand system
hand-bikes (arm ergometers), 49–50
hands-on therapy, 1, 2, 4, 6, 24–25, 69, 70, 71,
        78
Harvard University, 19, 34
HDL (high-density lipoprotein) cholesterol, 42,
        49
Healing Back Pain (Sarno), 32
health-care system, 237
heart disease, 41, 49
herniations, 7, 18, 87–88, 89, 143, 148, 172, 173,
        177–78, 238
hip, 169–96
    aging and, 177
    capsule of, 170, 172, 179
    cartilage of, 235
    damage to, 18
    dysfunction of, 177
    exercises for, 183–96
    flexors of, 161, 172, 174–75
    flexor tendinitis of, 174–75
    fractures of, 17, 46
    groin pain and, 171, 173–74, 177–79
    impingement of, 173, 177, 178, 180
    injury of, 169
    as joint, *see* joints
    movements of, 182
    osteoarthritis in, 181
    pain in, 19, 170, 171, 174–81
    pelvis and, 174
    reparation of, 178
    replacements of, 19, 66, 170, 178, 180
    resurfacing of, 180
    rotator muscles of, 148, 176
    socket of, 170, 171, 180, 235
hormones, 13, 17, 34, 40, 43, 150
Hospital for Special Surgery, 2, 43, 45, 87, 126,
        129, 149, 238
human evolution, 16, 34, 79–80, 102, 124–25, 179
humerus, 103, 104, 106, 110, 111, 126
hydration, 44–45

iliacus, 172, *197*
iliopsoas, 145, 172, 174, 175
iliopsoas tendon, 179
iliotibial (IT) band, *169,* 179, *197,* 199, 201, 210,
        211, 212
iliotibial band pain syndrome, 201
illness behavior, 30–31
immune system, 14, 40

inflammation:
    of bursas, 105–6
    corticosteroid injections and, 87, 89, 201
    friction as cause of, 24
    healing process and, 24
    injuries and, 130
    of joints, 5
    of muscles, *see* muscles, inflammation and
        irritation of
    omega-3 and, 38, 41, 47
    as problem, 24
infraspinatus, *102,* 104, 115, 119, 120, 122
injuries:
    acute, 86
    to ankle, 214
    to cartilage, 38
    chronic, 20–21, 33, 82–85, 86, 125
    to disks, 18
    exercise and, 63
    focal chondral, 208
    to foot, 214
    healing of, 75
    to hip, 169
    imbalance, 127
    inflammation and, 24, 87, 130
    to joints, 3, 16, 18, 22, 111, 237
    to knee, 197, 198, 201, 202, 204, 206, 208
    lower-extremity, 214
    misdiagnosed, 22, 31
    to muscles, 20–24
    to neck, 81, 82–85, 86–87
    occupational, 21
    overuse, 125, 128, 132, 214, 217
    prevention strategy for, 64
    repetitive stress, 20–21, 125, 127, 130
    to rotator cuffs, 105, 107–8
    to spinal cord, 81, 144
    in sports, ix–x, 2, 3
    tendonosis and, 221
    traumatic, 2, 4, 17, 20, 21, 24, 86–87, 110
    whiplash, 86–87
    to wrists, 134
insertion, 14
insulin, 41
insulin system, 41
integrated system, body as, 2, 11, 25, 80–81, 103,
        126, 132, 173, 198, 214, 235
integrated system of joints, muscles and, body as
        living material, 14, 17
integrins, 25
intensity, exercise and, 50–52, 62–63, 65–66
internal obliques, 145
intracapsular ligament, 170, *170*
intrinsic muscles, 94

as not covered by insurance, 240
physical therapy combined with, 87, 90, 129, 144, 206
on scarred muscle tissue, 4, 132
for spine, 7, 151
surgery vs., 109, 126
therapeutic techniques of, 70–72, 171
marrow cells, 14
Massachusetts, University of, 34
massage therapy, 24
medial collateral ligament (MCL), 204
medial epicondyle, *124,* 127
medial epicondylitis (golfer's elbow), 127, 128
medial tibial stress syndrome (shin splints), 214
median nerve, 133
meditation exercises, 34, 37
Mediterranean, 40
meniscus, 7, 15, 18, 19, 143, 197, 199–200, 202–3, 205, 208, 238
menopause, 45
methionine, 47
middle deltoids, 121
middle trapezius, 119, 121
mind-body disciplines, 35–36
mind-body exercises, 34–37
mind vs. body, 29–37
"mini-knee" (unicompartmental knee replacement), 207
Minnesota Vikings, 220
MIT, 34
mitochondria, 14
monounsaturated fats, 41
mortise joint, 214
Morton's neuroma, 221
MRI, 2, 3, 6, 7, 19, 31, 81, 85, 87, 105, 106, 143, 146, 148, 177, 202, 203, 220, 238, 239
mucoprotein gel, 15
multifidii, *142*
muscles, 11–13, 19–20
  aging of, 19, 20
  agonist, 12, 14, 20, 73, 145, 147
  antagonist, 12, 14, 20, 73, 74, 128, 145, 147, 216
  complementary groups of, 66
  conditioning work for, 69, 106, 130
  contraction of, 5, 7, 148, 173, 221
  damage to, 3, 24
  deterioration and weakening of, 20, 21, 132
  dysfunction of, 3, 21, 22, 29
  elements of, 3, 12–14, *13,* 15, 19, 24, 30, 77
  endurance of, 20, 49

function of, 12, 44
imbalances of, 21, 49, 99, 127, 128
inflammation and irritation of, 3, 20, 21, 24, 69, 88, 107, 108, 125, 127, 129, 148, 149, 177–78, 179, 202, 217
injuries and pain of, 3, 20–24, 30, 32, 34, 35, 143, 149, 151, 169, 173, 216
integrated system of bones, joints and, *see* integrated system, body as
joints and, 22, 81, 179, 194
lengthening of, 3, 72, 158, 160, 173
misdiagnosed problems of, 22
nerve damage and, 21, 83, 133
pressure on, 87, 110, 148
proprioception and, 12, 84
referral patterns of, 23, *23*
restriction of, 22, 30, 32
scar tissue and, 2, 4, 19, 24, 86, 105–6, 108, 132, 204
as self-healing, 3, 24
self-treatment exercises for, *see* self-treatment exercises
as shock absorbers, 15, 19, 30, 73
spasms of, 30, 31, 33, 70, 83
straining (pulling) of, 20, 30, 71, 104, 105–6, 125, 127, 149, 215
strengthening of, *see* strength work
stress and, 29–37, 55, 173
tendons and, *see* tendons
tension in, 31, 33, 35, 174
therapy for, 3, 5, 24–25, 33, 41, 74, 78, 88, 129, 144, 148, 150, 151, 181, 215, 220, 234, 240, 242; *see also specific therapies*
as tight, 3, 21, 22, 24, 30, 32, 33, 69, 108, 127, 128, 133
see also specific muscles
muscular corset, 152
muscular dystrophy, 21
musculoskeletal system:
  cushioning of, 15
  damage to, 7
  evolution and, 16
  exercise for, 48, 53
  injuries of, 214, 220, 240
  maintaining health of, 38, 40, 45–47, 236
  problems of, 2, 6, 25, 33, 36, 125, 215, 234–35, 239
  psychological stress and, 4–5
  self-knowledge of, 237
  therapies and, 69, 72
Myofascial Release, 71, 240
myofibril, 13, *13*
myosin, 13

therapy vs., 7, 25, 150–51, 178–79, 203
on vertebrae and facets, 151
swimming, 49, 62, 63, 65, 66, 107
syndromes, *see specific syndromes*
synovial fluid, 15, 18, 48–49
systems, *see specific body systems*

tai chi, 36
talus, 214
tarsal tunnel, 216, 220
tarsal tunnel syndrome, 220
tendinitis, 22, 104, 107, 108, 128–29, 174–75
tendinous sheath, 198
tendonosis, 22, 129, 219, 221
tendons, *13*
    aging and, 107
    collagen fibers of, 15, 17, 22, 129, 219
    conditioning exercises for, 130, 220
    deterioration of, 22
    inflammation and irritation of, 127
    lengthening of, 72
    overstressed, 28
    pain due to, 22, 24, 110
    purpose of, 13, 103
    rupture of, 221
    scarring of, 129
    tears in, 18, 19, 103, 106, 108, 171, 198
    see also specific tendons
tennis-elbow (lateral epicondylitis), 22, 125, 127, 128–29, 219
tension headache (occipital neuralgia), 82, 83
tensor fasciae latae, *197,* 199
teres muscles, 118
    teres major, *102*
    teres minor, *102,* 104, 122
testosterone, 13
TheraCane, 153
therapy, surgery vs., 7, 25, 150–51, 178–79, 203
    see also specific therapies and techniques
thoracic spine, 80, 83, 145
tibia, 198, 199–200, 201, 203, 204, 205, 206, 214
tibialis anterior, *213,* 216, 223, 228
tibialis posterior, 216
tibial nerve, 220
tibial osteotomy, 207
Toomer, Amani, x, 220–21
Torres, Dara, 20
trans fats, 41, 44
trapezius muscles, *23, 79,* 94, 95, 104, 115, 118, 119, 121
trauma surgeons, 234
Travell, Janet, 25
treadmill, 53, 61
treatment sticks, 5, 153

triceps, 14, *102,* 114, 118, 127, 128
Trigger Point Therapy, 24–25, 71, 72, 236, 240
trochanteric bursitis, 179

ulna, 126, 134
ulnar nerve, 127, 133
ulnar nerve entrapment, 133
unicompartmental knee replacement, 207
upper trapezius muscles, *23, 79,* 94, 95, 104, 115, 121

vastus intermedius, *197,* 199
vastus lateralis, *197,* 199, 200, 210
vastus medialis, *197,* 199, 200
vertebrae, 7, 15, 17, 80, 81, 82, 87, 88, 89, 143, 148, 150, 151, 159
vitamin D, 38, 45–46
vitamins, 41
volumetrics, 41

walking, 30, 50, 62, 151
warm-up, for exercise, 53
weight, body, *see* body weight
weighted ball, 60
weight lifting, 78
weight machines, 73
weights:
    ankle, 193
    hand, 121, 122, 123, 140, 141
Weill Cornell Medical College, 2
whiplash injury, 86–87
Women's Sports Medicine Center, 43
wood chop exercise, 60, *61*
wrist:
    extension of, 141
    extra motion of, 128
    fracturing of, 134
    injury to, 134
    motions of, 135
    overuse injuries of, 125
    pain in, 125
    protection of, 131
    splints for, 132, 133, 134
    spraining of, 134
    versatility of, 126
    see also elbow/wrist/hand system; forearm
wrist extensor muscles, 75

X-rays, 2, 6, 7, 31, 81, 134, 181, 202, 239

yoga, 35–36, 54, 176

Zinn, Sister Carol, 202
Zyflamend, 47